Symposia in Neuroscience, Volume 7

NEURONAL PLASTICITY
AND TROPHIC FACTORS

Symposia in Neuroscience

Series editors

GIOVANNI BIGGIO
Professor of Pharmacology
School of Biology
University of Cagliari
Cagliari, Italy

ERMINIO COSTA
Director, Fidia Georgetown
Institute for the Neurosciences FGIN
Washington D.C., 20007, USA

SYMPOSIA IN NEUROSCIENCE
Volume 7

NEURONAL PLASTICITY AND TROPHIC FACTORS

Edited by

Giovanni Biggio
Professor of Pharmacology
School of Biology
University of Cagliari
Cagliari, Italy

Pier Franco Spano
Professor of Pharmacology
School of Medicine
University of Brescia
Brescia, Italy

Gino Toffano
Director
FIDIA Research Laboratories
Abano Terme
Padova, Italy

Stanley H. Appel
Professor of Neurology
Baylor College of Medicine
Texas Medical Center
Houston, Texas

Gian Luigi Gessa
Professor of Pharmacology
School of Medicine
University of Cagliari
Cagliari, Italy

FIDIA
RESEARCH
SERIES

LIVIANA PRESS
Italy

SPRINGER VERLAG
Berlin - Heidelberg
New York - Tokyo

FIDIA RESEARCH SERIES

An open-end series of publications on international biomedical research, with special emphasis on the neurosciences, published by LIVIANA Press, Padova, Italy, in cooperation with FIDIA Research Labs, Abano Terme, Italy.

The series will be devoted to advances in basic and clinical research in the neurosciences and other fields.

The aim of the series is the rapid and worldwide dissemination of up-to-date, interdisciplinary data as presented at selected international scientific meetings and study groups.

Each volume is published under the editorial responsibility of scientists chosen by organizing committees of the meetings on the basis of their active involvement in the research of the field concerned.

DISTRIBUTION

Sole distribution rights outside Italy granted to Springer - Verlag.
All orders for the Fidia Research Series should be sent to the following addresses

Italy:
LIVIANA EDITRICE S.p.A. - Via Luigi Dottesio, 1, 35138 Padova, Italia

North America:
SPRINGER - VERLAG New York, Inc. - 175 Fifth Avenue, New York, N.Y. 10010, USA

Japan:
SPRINGER - VERLAG - 37-3 Hongo 3-chome, Bunkyo-Ku, Tokyo 113, Japan

Rest of the World:
SPRINGER - VERLAG Berlin - Heidelberger Platz 3, 1000 Berlin 33, FRG

Printed in Italy

ISBN   88-7675-529-2   Liviana Editrice
ISBN   3-540-96796-6   Springer - Verlag Berlin Heidelberg New York Tokyo
ISBN   0-387-96796-6   Springer - Verlag New York Heidelberg Berlin Tokyo

---

LIVIANA Editrice S.p.A. - via Luigi Dottesio 1, 35138, Padova, Italy.

PREFACE

Among the most exciting advances in our understanding of the brain has been the recognition of the role of neuronal plasticity and trophic factors in brain growth, development, and the repair of injury.

Neurotrophic factors play a key role in these processes by influencing information transfer between neurons. The seminal work of Rita Levi Montalcini established the importance of nerve growth factor (NGF) as a target-derived polipeptide whose retrograde effects enhance neuronal growth and development. By analogy with NGF, a number of other growth factors have been demonstrated to influence neuronal development in vitro. The key themes in neurotrophic factor research are discussed in the present symposium. The cellular levels and localization of NGF on gene expression are included.

Other putative neurotrophic factors such as basic fibroblast growth factor, epithelial growth factor, striatal derived neurotrophic factor, and serum factors enhancing growth of cerebellar granule cells, are also discussed. Finally, the ability of ganglioside as well as NGF to prevent cholinergic degeneration in vivo, the mechanisms of plasticity in short and long term learning and effects of nerve grafts on regrowth of CNS neurons are presented.

The investigations included in this volume serve to underscore the tremendous progress that has been made in our understanding of neuronal growth and development and the hope that such progress can be translated into meaningful therapeutic strategies for patients afflicted with severe neurological deficits.

Stanley H. Appel, M.D.
Houston, December 1987

ACKNOWLEDGEMENT

This volume presents the proceedings of the 5th Capo Boi Conference on Neuroscience held at Villasimius, Italy, in May 1987. This conference was made possible by the generous support given by the FIDIA Research Laboratories (Abano Terme).

The Editors would like to take this opportunity to express their gratitude and appreciation.

CONTENTS

S.H. Appel, J.R. Bostwick, L.J. Haverkamp, J.L. McManaman, *Multiple trophic factors influence neuronal cholinergic activity* 1

R.A. Bradshaw, M. Blaber, K. Cavanaugh, D.D. Eveleth, P.J. Isackson, H.I. Kornblum, F. Leslie, R.S. Morrison, M. Schwarz, A. Sharma, *Neurotrophic factors of the central nervous system: synthesis and activities* 9

S. Korsching, R. Heumann, A.M. Davies, H. Thoenen, *Levels of nerve growth factor and its mRNA during development and regeneration of the peripheral nervous system* 23

C.E. Bandtlow, R. Heumann, M.E. Schwab, H. Thoenen, *Cellular localization of nerve growth factor synthesis in various organs of the peripheral nervous system* 35

A. Levi, R. Possenti, J. Eldridge, B.M. Paterson, *Studies on a gene sequence whose expression is regulated by NGF in PC12 cells* 45

D. Gospodarowicz, N. Ferrara, *The control of cell growth and differentiation by fibroblast growth factor* 53

R.E. Rydel, L.A. Greene, *8-substituted cAMP analogs can replace the NGF requirement of cultured rat sympathetic and sensory neurons: evidence for parallel neurotrophic pathways* 73

G. Ferrari, C. Soranzo, L. Callegaro, R. Dal Toso, D. Benvegnú, G. Toffano, A. Leon, *Characterization and purification of a striatal-derived neuronotrophic factor (SDNF)* 87

D. Mercanti, M.T. Ciotti, P. Calissano, *A serum factor inducing neurite outgrowth and cell adhesion in cerebellar granule cells* 95

A.C. Cuello, E.P. Pioro, D. Maysinger, L. Garofalo, P.C. Tagari, *Application of gangliosides, nerve growth factor and brain transplants to prevent cholinergic degeneration in the central nervous system* 105

G.M. Bray, M.P. Villegas-Pérez, M. Vidal-Sanz, A.J. Aguayo, *Effects of peripheral nerve grafts on the survival and regrowth of axotomized CNS neurons* 121

VIII

M. Brunelli, L. Colombaioni, G. Traina, *Mechanisms of plasticity in short and long term learning process in invertebrates* 129

Plenary Lecture on:
Research strategies for the therapy of aging brain

G. Pepeu, I. Marconcini Pepeu 139

Contributors 149

Subject Index 153

Neuronal Plasticity and Trophic Factors
G. Biggio, P.F. Spano, G. Toffano, S.H. Appel, G.L. Gessa (eds.)
Fidia Research Series, Symposia in Neuroscience VII
Liviana Press, Padova © 1988

MULTIPLE TROPHIC FACTORS INFLUENCE NEURONAL CHOLINERGIC ACTIVITY

**Stanley H. Appel, James R. Bostwick,
Lanny J. Haverkamp and James L. McManaman**

Department of Neurology, Baylor College of Medicine,
Houston, Texas 77030, USA

INTRODUCTION

The development and maintenance of neurons is under multiple levels of interacting controls, including functional activity, intrinsic programs for differentiation, contact-mediated cellular interactions, and diffusible signals from target and support cells. In our attempt to understand the nature of diffusible signals, we have concentrated our efforts on trophic factors which are released by neural target tissues and exert a retrograde influence on neuronal growth and development. The best example of such a trophic factor is Nerve Growth Factor. The active moiety, a 26,500 dalton beta dimer, has been purified (Bocchini and Angeletti, 1969), sequenced (Angeletti et al., 1973) and cloned (Scott et al., 1983; Ullrich et al., 1983). NGF plays a critical role in the development and maintenance of the sympathetic and sensory nervous systems. Both NGF and its RNA are first detected in target tissue at the time that innervating neurons reach the target (Davies et al., 1987) and both increase significantly over the next several days (Davies et al., 1987). Subsequently, NGF is found in the innervating ganglia, having interacted with specific surface receptors on axon terminals, and having passed by retrograde axonal transport to cell bodies (Thoenen and Barde, 1980). In accord with this interpretation is the absence of NGF mRNA in the cell bodies of innervating neurons despite the presence of significant NGF levels (Davies et al., 1987).

The most cogent evidence for the biological role of NGF is the deleterious effect of anti-NGF antibodies on sympathetic and sensory neurons when administered to developing animals. Prenatal exposure to anti-NGF antibodies markedly impairs sensory neuron development (Gorin and Johnson, 1979) while both prenatal and early postnatal administration produce profound immunosympathectomy (Cohen, 1960; Levi-Montalcini and Booker, 1960).

Recent studies have suggested that NGF may also play a significant role in development of neurons within the CNS. NGF and its mRNA are present in cortex and hippocampus (Large et al., 1986; Whittemore et al., 1986; Shelton and Reichardt, 1986), while NGF receptors (Richardson et al., 1986) and NGF itself are found in the cholinergic neurons of the nucleus basalis and the medial septal nucleus, which project to the cortex and hippocampus respectively (Schwab et al., 1979; Seiler and Schwab, 1984; Whittemore et al., 1986). Antibodies to NGF clearly block actions of NGF *in vitro* in medial septal explants (Bostwick et al., 1987), but administration of anti-NGF antibodies *in vivo* appears to have minimal effects (Gnahn et al., 1983). The inability of anti-NGF antibodies to influence septal-hippocampal cholinergic development has been attributed to failure of the antibodies to reach the appropriate intracellular target sites. Why such impenetrability should be present within the CNS but not within sensory and sympathetic ganglia is not clear. One possibility is that while anti-NGF antibodies are equally accessible to septal, sensory, and sympathetic neurons, central cholinergic development depends not upon a single factor such as NGF, but upon multiple factors. Elimination of a single factor may thus have far fewer deleterious effects in the CNS than are seen in peripheral ganglia.

RESULTS AND DISCUSSION

By analogy with NGF, we anticipated that other trophic factors from peripheral and control target tissues would have effects on development and regeneration. Our own laboratories initially focused on identifying a single factor from muscle which could promote motor neuron survival, neurite elongation, and enhancement of cholinergic activity. This moiety was unlikely to be NGF itself since NGF and anti-NGF antibodies have no known influence on differentiation of cultured ventral horn cells. In order to define the different neurons of the ventral horn, three different techniques were employed.

Neurons were defined by their specific interaction with tetanus toxin *in vitro*. Motor neurons were also defined as those cells whose axons extend to the periphery and can retrogradely transport wheat germ agglutinin-lucifer yellow to the cell body (Fig. 1). The marker was retained by those cells during dissection, dissociation, and subsequent culturing on polylysine coated dishes. Such cells comprised 1.3% of the tetanus toxin-labeled cells in untreated cultures after four days. Cholinergic neurons were defined by their ability to stain with the monoclonal antibody to choline acetyltransferase linked to horseradish peroxidase (Fig. 2). Such cells comprised approximately 8% of cells after 4.5 days in culture.

These techniques permitted us to define the factors derived from muscle extracts which influence survival and neurite elongation of motor and non-motor neurons and to define those factors which enhance acetylcholine synthesis and choline acetyltransferase

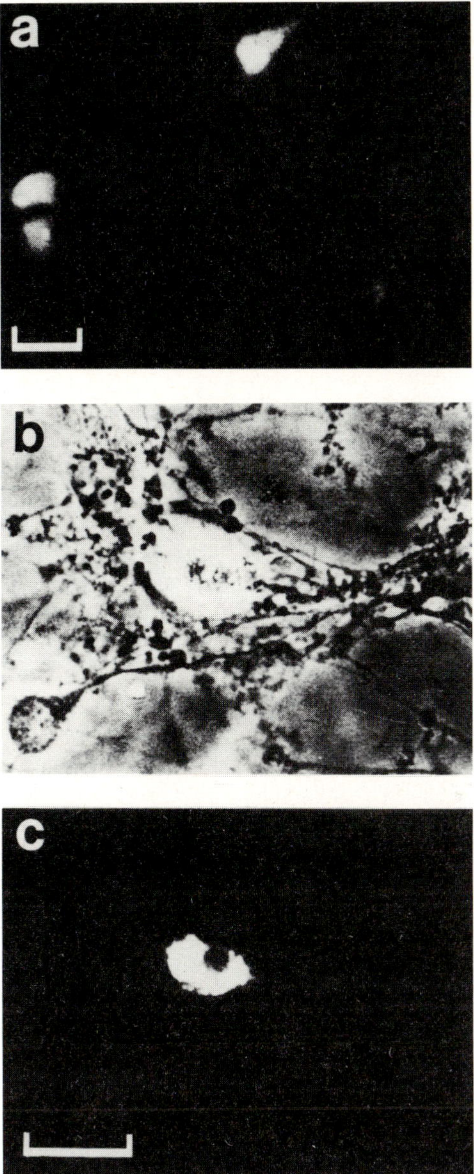

Figure 1. Use of WGA-LY in motoneuron visualization. 75-100 µg of labeled WGA was injected *in situ* into rat 14 d embryo hindlimbs. After a 4 hr incubation at 30°C, spinal cords were removed from the embryos, and prepared as described in the text. a. Portion of anterior horn slice taken from thoracolumbar region of embryonic cord. Individual cells in the slice are labeled with the probe. No staining was observed in the dorsal portion of the spinal cord ($\times 500$); b. Phase-contrast; and c. Fluorescence micrographs of WGA-LY-labeled cells, raised in culture for 4 days in the presence of 200 µg muscle extract/ml culture medium ($\times 800$). Bars, 20 µm. (Smith et al., 1986).

4

activity. A 35,000 dalton glycoprotein was found to influence neurite extension from both motor neurons and non-motor neurons. This acidic glycoprotein had no influence on either acetylcholine synthesis or choline acetyltransferase activity. It had no effect on dorsal horn cells or dorsal root ganglia.

In our initial studies two different muscle fractions, a 1200-1500 dalton and 56,000 dalton constituent, were found to enhance acetylcholine synthesis. At saturating doses these moieties were additive to one another in restoring the full cholinergic enhancing potential of the original muscle extract. The 1500 dalton constituent enhanced survival of motor neurons but had no effect on non-motor neurons, while the 56,000 dalton protein had no effect on neuronal survival but did enhance selective process outgrowth and elongation as well as acetylcholine synthesis in motor neurons.

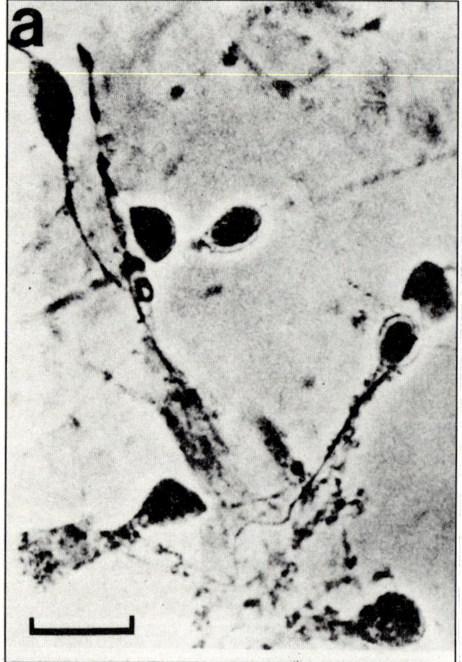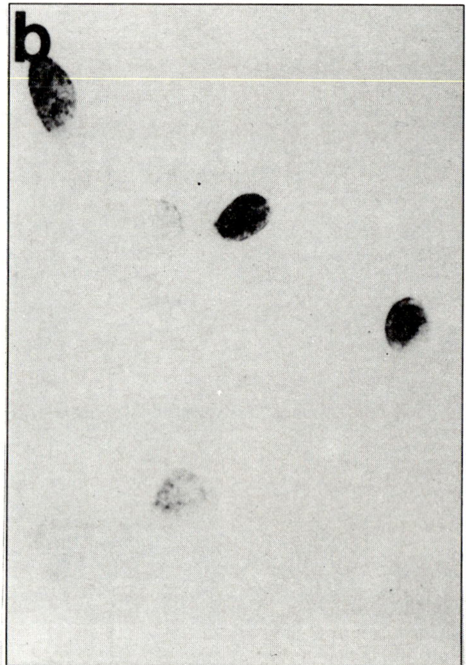

Figure 2. Phase-contrast (a) and bright-field (b) photomicrographs depicting CAT antibody-labeling cells. Cells are visually assayed for diaminobenzidene reaction product by subjectively assigning each cell in random microscopic fields to one of four categories: (1) heavy or dense labeling, (2) moderate labeling, (3) light or indeterminate labeling, and (4) no labeling. *Heavily stained and moderately stained cells* are grouped together as "positively labeled", while *unstained and indeterminately stained cells* are defined as "not labeled". By such subjective analysis, two heavily labeled and one moderately labeled CAT-staining cells are extending processes in this image, made after 5 d in the presence of 400 μg crude muscle extract/ml culture medium. Note the presence of two lightly stained and two non-reactive neuron-like cells, together with several unstained non-neuronal cells (× 100). Bar, 20 μm. (Smith et al., 1986).

Since these studies were carried out with cultured rat ventral horn cells, it is not clear whether all such factors will influence ventral spinal cord development *in vivo*. In development of the motor neuron *in vivo* axon elongation to the periphery occurs prior to neuronal cell death, while marked enhancement of cholinergic activity occurs subsequent to both events. The developmental sequence could certainly be fostered by a single factor, but if our *in vitro* data are applicable *in vivo*, it is more likely that multiple factors play carefully and precisely orchestrated roles in motor neuron development.

Within the central nervous system, multiple factors also appear to participate in neuronal development. Our own efforts have focused on cholinergic neurons of the medial septum. A 1000 dalton constituent (C-CTF) derived from hippocampus and cortex enhances acetylcholine synthesis and to a lesser extent choline acetyltransferase activity in explants of 16-day-old rat medial septum. In this same system, NGF enhances choline acetyltransferase activity yet has minimal effects on acetylcholine synthesis activity. When concentrations of each factor which maximally enhance choline acetyltransferase activity are simultaneously applied in culture, there is an additive and occasionally a synergistic effect. The 1000 dalton moiety is clearly not a breakdown product of NGF, since no small peptide derived from NGF is known to have trophic activity, and antibodies to NGF have no effect on the activity of the 1000 dalton constituent. Neither NGF nor the 1000 dalton constituent appear to enhance choline uptake in a significant fashion. However, C-CTF promotes a greater conversion of the incorporated choline into acetylcholine than does NGF, even though NGF has the greater stimulatory effect on choline acetyltransferase activity. Although the mechanisms of stimulation of CAT activity cannot be defined by these data, NGF and C-CTF appear to act on different pathways.

Recently another growth factor has been demonstrated to influence CNS neurons *in vitro*. Basic fibroblast growth factor is a 16,000 dalton polypeptide isolated from pituitary and brain. This factor stimulates angiogenesis *in vivo* (Esch et al., 1985) and is mitogenic for many different cell types, including glia (Pruss et al., 1981). Basic FGF has been reported to enhance survival and neurite elongation in cultures of hippocampal neurons (Walicke et al., 1986). In this report, neurons were derived from 18-day-old rat embryos, plated on plastic, or on laminin-coated plastic, and maintained continuously in defined serum-free culture conditions. Concentrations of basic FGF from 10-100 pg/ml were able to enhance neuronal survival while slightly higher concentrations enhanced neurite outgrowth. Another study has documented that basic FGF promotes the elaboration of neurites and the survival of rat cortical neurons when the FGF is added after the cells have been grown for 18 hours in 10% fetal bovine serum and cytosine arabinoside, and are then switched to serum-free defined medium (Morrison et al., 1986). Under these conditions, other growth factors such as thrombin, platelet-derived growth factor, beta NGF, and interleukin 2 had no effects. Neither of these studies are able to indicate whether basic FGF acts directly on a neuronal receptor, or indirectly by action on glia. Both reports reject the likely participation of glia because of the relatively small population of glia present. Nevertheless, since both laminin and glial conditioned medium can influence neuronal viability *in vitro* (Barde et al., 1978; Pixley and Cotman, 1986), effects of glia and extracellular matrix must be considered. The lack of direct data demonstrating neuronal effects precludes a more definitive statement.

In our laboratory we have found basic FGF to enhance acetylcholine synthesis in

6

cultured medial septal explants (Fig. 3). Basic FGF at doses of 15 ng/ml was found to enhance acetylcholine synthesis half as effectively as C-CTF. In this set of experiments, NGF enhanced acetylcholine synthesis. The combination of NGF and C-CTF, however, had a more marked stimulatory effect than any combination of either factor with basic FGF, and addition of all three factors to culture showed no increase over that seen with C-CTF and NGF alone. Whether basic FGF enhances acetylcholine synthesis activity by an effect on neuronal differentiation, and whether such effects are exerted directly or indirectly, by actions on glia, is not presently clear. At the very least, the additive effects of the factors suggest different mechanisms of action, and similarly the existence of different mechanisms imply the action of diverse trophic influences.

With the use of *in vivo* labeling of motor neurons with wheat germ agglutinin-lucifer yellow, and *in vitro* choline acetyltransferase immunohistochemistry, effects of muscle-derived factors on neuronal survival can be distinguished from effects on cholinergic activity. However, retrograde labeling techniques are difficult to apply to the embryonic brain and choline acetyltransferase immunohistochemistry cannot be used *per se* to distinguish reliably between effects on survival and effects on enhancement of cholinergic activity. It is clear that trophic factors can enhance CAT activity. What is not clear is whether the primary effect is directly on neuronal survival, or on process

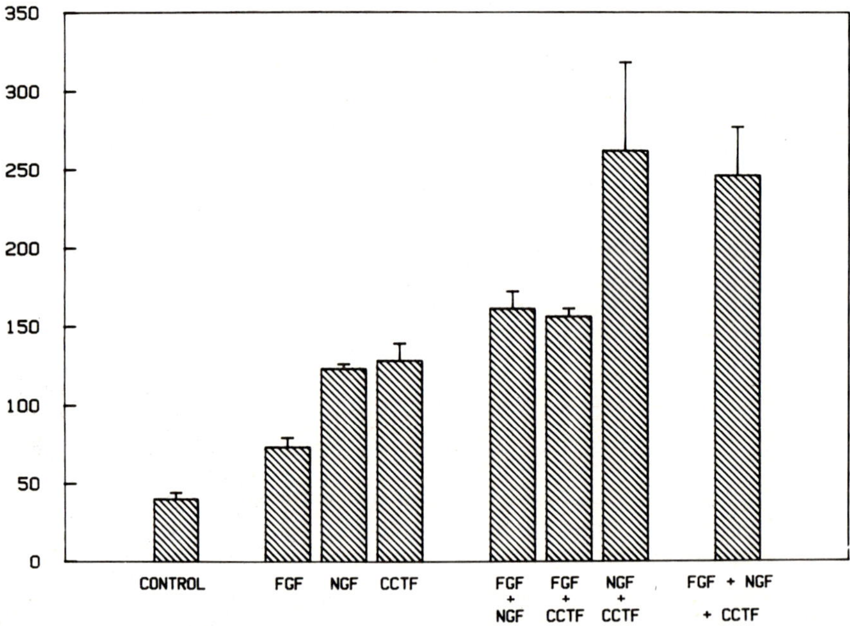

Figure 3. Stimulation of acetylcholine synthesis by FGF, NGF and CCTF in the medial septal explant culture. Explant cultures were prepared, maintained, and assayed as described previously (Bostwick et al., 1987). Additions of trophic factors were made on culture days 2 and 8 and Ach synthesis was assayed on day 8. Concentrations of factors were as follows: FGF, 15 ng/ml:NGF, 50 ng/ml: CCTF, 10 mg/ml (estimate for protein by fluorescein assay).

elongation or cholinergic differentiation, or whether the effect is indirectly on neurons by an action in glia. Any of these pathways would lead to the same end point of enhanced CAT activity or enhanced acetylcholine synthesis. Nevertheless, it is clear that in both the development of motor neurons as well as in the development of medial septum neurons *in vitro*, multiple factors play a meaningful role.

In the present conference the contribution by Rydel and Greene suggests that in the sympathetic and sensory systems, a mechanism unresponsive to NGF, namely cyclic AMP-dependent protein kinases, can promote long-term neuronal survival and neurite outgrowth. Thus, even in NGF-responsive neurons multiple factors may play a significant role in fostering neuronal development.

CONCLUSION

These experiments document the complexity of neuronal development and response to injury and the multiplicity of developmental stages. Each of the developmental stages and each aspect of regeneration may be differentially influenced by different factors. The end point of differentiation (e.g., ACh synthesis) or regeneration (e.g., axon regeneration) may not reflect the trophic action of a single factor. NGF is clearly a trophic factor for septal neurons but does not affect the end point of differentiation, ACh synthesis, although it does influence CAT activity. Thus a component of cholinergic differentiation, namely CAT, must be assayed to clearly demonstrate NGF's effect. Similarly, a component of the response to injury (e.g., transmitter levels, lysosomal enzymes, cell body transmitter receptors, ODC, actin, etc.) might be more likely to reflect a factor's trophic effect than will the end point of regeneration.

ACKNOWLEDGMENT

We are grateful to the Harkins Foundation Fund for Alzheimer's disease and the Robert J. Kleberg and Helen C. Kleberg Foundation, for support of these studies.

REFERENCES

Angeletti RH, Mercanti D, Bradshaw RA (1973a) Amino acid sequences of mouse 2.5S nerve growth factor. I. Isolation and characterization of the soluble tryptic and chymotryptic peptides. Biochemistry 12:90-100.

Angeletti RH, Hermodson MA, Bradshaw RA (1973b) Amino acid sequences of mouse 2.5S nerve growth factor. II. Isolation and characterization of the thermolytic and peptic peptides and the complete covalent structure. Biochemistry 12:100-115.

Barde YA, Lindsay RM, Monard D, Thoenen H (1978) New factor released by cultured glioma cells supporting survival and growth of sensory neurons. Nature London 274:818.

Bocchini V, Angeletti PU (1969) The nerve growth factor: purification as a 30,000-molecular-weight protein. Proc Natl Acad Sci USA 64:787-794.

Bostwick JR, Appel SH, Perez-Polo JR (1987) Distinct influences of nerve growth factor and a central cholinergic trophic factor on medial septal explants. Brain Research 422:92-98.

Cohen S (1960) Purification of a nerve-growth promoting protein from the mouse salivary gland and its neurocytotoxic antiserum. Proc Natl Acad Sci USA 46:301-311.

Davies AM, Bandtlow C, Heumann R, Korsching S, Rohrer H, Thoenen H (1987) Timing and site of nerve growth factor synthesis in developing skin in relation to innervation and expression of the receptor. Nature 326:353-358.

Esch F, Baird A, Ling N, Veno N, Hill F, Denoroy L, Klepper R, Gospodarowicz D, Bohlen P, Guillemin R (1985) Primary structure of bovine pituitary basic fibroblast growth factor (FGF) and comparison with the amino terminal sequence of bovine brain acidic FGF. Proc Natl Acad Sci USA 82:6507-6511.

Gnahn H, Hefti F, Heumann R, Schwab ME, Thoenen H (1983) NGF-mediated increase of choline acetyltransferase (ChAT) in the neonatal rat forebrain: Evidence for a physiological role of NGF in the brain? Dev Brain Res 9:45-52.

Gorin PD, Johnson EM (1979) Experimental autoimmune model of nerve growth factor deprivation: Effects on developing peripheral sympathetic and sensory neurons. Proc Natl Acad Sci USA 76:5382-5386.

Large TH, Bodary SC, Clegg DO, Weskamp G, Otten U, Reichardt LF (1986) Nerve growth factor gene expression in the developing rat brain. Science 234:352-355.

Levi-Montalcini R, Booker B (1960) Destruction of the sympathetic ganglia in mammals by an antiserum to the nerve growth promoting factor. Proc Natl Acad Sci USA 46:384-391.

Morrison RS, Sharma A, de Vellis J, Bradshaw RA (1986) Basic fibroblast growth factor supports the survival of cerebral cortical neurons in primary culture. Proc Natl Acad Sci USA 83:7537-7541.

Pixley SK, Cotman CW (1986) Laminin supports short-term survival of rat septal neurons in low density, serum-free cultures. J Neurosci Res 15:1-17.

Pruss RM, Bartlett PF, Gaurilovic J, Lisak RP, Rattray S (1981) Mitogens for glial cells: A comparison of the response of cultured astrocytes, oligodendrocytes and Schwann cells. Dev Brain Res 2:19-35.

Richardson PM, Verge Issa VMK, Riopelle RJ (1986) Distribution of neuronal receptors for nerve growth factor in the rat. J Neurosci 6(8):2313-2321.

Schwab ME, Otten U, Agid Y, Thoenen H (1979) Nerve growth factor (NGF) in the rat CNF: Absence of specific retrograde axonal transport and tyrosine hydroxylase induction in locus coeruleus and substantia nigra. Brain Res 168(3):473-483.

Scott J, Selby M, Urdea M, Quiroga M, Bell GI, Rutter WJ (1983) Isolation and nucleotide sequence of a cDNA encoding the precursor of mouse nerve growth factor. Nature 302:538-540.

Seiler M, Schwab ME (1984) Specific retrograde transport of nerve growth factor (NGF) from neocortex to nucleus basalis in the rat. Brain Res 300:33-39.

Shelton DL, Reichardt LF (1986) Studies on the expression of the β nerve growth factor (NGF) gene in the central nervous system: Level and regional distribution of NGF mRNA suggest that NGF functions as a trophic factor for several distinct populations of neurons. Proc Natl Acad Sci USA 83:2714-2718.

Smith RG, Vaca K, McManaman J, Appel SH (1986) Selective effects of skeletal muscle extract fractions on motoneuron development in vitro. J Neurosci 6 (20): 439-447.

Thoenen A, Barde YA (1980) Physiology of nerve growth factor. Physiol Rev 60:1284-1335.

Ullrich A, Gray A, Berman C, Dull TJ (1983) Human beta-nerve growth factor gene sequence highly homologous to that of mouse. Nature 303:821-825.

Walicke P, Cowan WM, Veno N (1986) Fibroblast growth factor promotes survival of dissociated hippocampal neurons and enhances neurite extension. Proc Natl Acad Sci USA 83:7537-7541.

Whittemore SR, Ebendal T, Larkfors L, Olson L, Seiger A, Stromberg, Persson H (1986) Developmental and regional expression of B nerve growth factor messenger RNA and protein in the rat central nervous system. Proc Natl Acad Sci USA 83:817-821.

Neuronal Plasticity and Trophic Factors
G. Biggio, P.F. Spano, G. Toffano, S.H. Appel, G.L. Gessa (eds.)
Fidia Research Series, Symposia in Neuroscience VII
Liviana Press, Padova © 1988

NEUROTROPHIC FACTORS OF THE CENTRAL NERVOUS SYSTEM: SYNTHESIS AND ACTIVITIES

Ralph A. Bradshaw[1], Michael Blaber[1], Kathleen Cavanaugh[1], David D. Eveleth[1], Paul J. Isackson[1,2], Harley I. Kornblum[3], Frances Leslie[3], Richard S. Morrison[1], Martin Schwarz[1] and Arun Sharma[1]

Departments of [1]Biological Chemistry, [2]Anatomy and Neurobiology and [3]Pharmacology, California College of Medicine, University of California, Irvine, CA 92717, USA

INTRODUCTION

Although the mechanisms underlying the development and maintenance of neurons is incompletely understood, substantial evidence has accumulated suggesting that neurotrophic factors are central to these processes (Barde et al., 1983; Berg, 1984). The interaction of nerve growth factor (NGF)[1] with various peripheral neurons has been pivotal in elucidating this concept (Levi-Montalcini, 1987). In general, these factors, which are largely if not exclusively polypeptides, interact with receptors located in the plasma membrane of the neuron to affect the responses necessary to sustain viability. Depending on the stage of development or other environmental intrusions, the sites of synthesis are confined to neuronal targets and/or support (glial) cells (Rush, 1984;

Abbreviations used: NGF-α, -β and -γ: α, β and γ subunits of mouse nerve growth factor, 7S NGF: high molecular weight complex of mouse nerve growth factor, EGF: epidermal growth factor, HMW-EGF: high molecular weight epidermal growth factor, EGF-BP: epidermal growth factor binding protein, TGF-α: transforming growth factor-α, bFGF: basic fibroblast growth factor.
Present addresses: Richard S. Morrison: Department of Neurological Surgery, Montefiore Hospital, Bronx, NY 10467, USA; Arun Sharma: Department of Physiology, California College of Medicine, University of California, Irvine, CA 92717, USA.

Davies et al., 1987). The receptor molecules may be concentrated in the pre-synaptic membrane or they can be more widely distributed along axons and on cell bodies (Greene and Shooter, 1980). In mature neurons, the binding at the presynaptic membrane leads to internalization and retrograde axonal transport; however, the importance of this event mechanistically is still unknown (James and Bradshaw, 1984).

The characterization of neurotrophic factors, as a group, has proceeded only slowly. By analogy with NGF, it has been generally assumed that there exists a substantial subgroup of polypeptide growth factors, with suitable variety to accomodate the diversity of neuronal elements within the CNS (Berg, 1984). Interestingly, the most significant recent advances in identifying such factors have come from the realization that many well-known polypeptide growth factors, recognized mainly for their mitogenic properties on various target cells, can also act, at least *in vitro*, as neuronotrophic agents on cultured CNS neurons. These findings follow the well established pattern of multiple usage of peptides, commonly acting in various endocrine capacities, on the one hand, and in apparently different ways in the brain, on the other. Even NGF, whose activities in the CNS identified in earlier studies lacked molecular and cellular correlations (Berger et al., 1973; Hart et al., 1978; Lewis et al., 1979), has now been shown to interact in a functionally significant fashion with cholinergic neurons in the CNS (Gnahn et al., 1983; Honegger and Lenoir, 1983; Hefti et al., 1984; 1985; Mobley et al., 1985; Fischer et al., 1987).

Two polypeptide growth factors that have been found to support CNS neuronal preparations are epidermal growth factor (EGF) and basic fibroblast growth factor (bFGF) (Walicke et al., 1986; Morrison et al., 1986; 1987). The latter is found in significant concentrations in the brain (and pituitary) as well as elsewhere (Gospadarowicz et al., 1984; Lobb et al., 1986). The distribution of EGF in the CNS is apparently much more limited (Fallon et al., 1984) and somewhat more controversial (Probstmeier and Schachner, 1986). Interestingly, these same two factors, along with NGF, also effect the clonal transformed cell line PC12 derived from a rat pheochromocytoma, albeit in different ways (Greene and Tischler, 1982). In this article, we consider aspects of both the synthesis and neurotrophic function of these factors.

BIOSYNTHESIS

NGF and EGF Production in the Mouse Submandibular Gland

From analysis of cDNA clones, the mature forms of the hormonally-active subunits of NGF and EGF are excised from considerably larger precursor molecules in the mouse submandibular gland and in probably most, if not all, other sites of synthesis as well (Scott et al., 1983a; 1983b; Gray et al., 1983; Ullrich et al., 1983). In each case, this involves a minimum of two proteolytic cleavages (Fig. 1). With NGF, the amino terminal serine of the β-subunit is formed by an as yet unidentified protease that cleaves to the carboxyl side of a pair of basic residues (Lys-Arg). A second hydrolysis results in the removal of a dipeptide, Arg-Gly, leaving a C-terminal arginine residue on the mature protein. In contrast, single arginine residues form both activation sites for the production of mature EGF; the excised pieces are potentially much greater in size than those released from the NGF precursor.

Both hormones occur in the gland (or saliva) as complexes containing other subunits. The NGF complex (7S NGF) contains two other polypeptides (2 copies each) while the EGF complex (HMW-EGF) has only one (also 2 copies). One of the NGF subunits (γ) and the EGF-binding protein (EGF-BP) are active serine proteases with a strong preference for arginine bonds (Greene et al., 1968; Taylor et al., 1974). The third subunit (NGF-α) is rather similar in primary structure to NGF-γ and EGF-BP but it is catalytically inactive, presumably as the result of a number of mutations at the amino terminus and near the potential active site serine (Isackson et al., 1984). The complete amino acid sequence of mouse NGF-γ was determined directly (Thomas et al., 1981) and subsequently by cDNA sequence analysis (Ullrich et al., 1984). In contrast only partial protein sequences were determined for NGF-α (Isackson and Bradshaw, 1984; Ronne et al., 1984) and EGF-BP (Anundi et al., 1982). The complete sequences of both precursors were deduced from cloned cDNA molecules (Isackson et al., 1984; Blaber et al., 1987).

The identification of the protein corresponding to EGF-BP proved to be challenging, owing in large part to the considerable number of closely related proteases found in the mouse submandibular gland (Mason et al., 1983). This complex consists of both expressed and pseudo genes (Evans et al., 1987) and all are sequentially related to

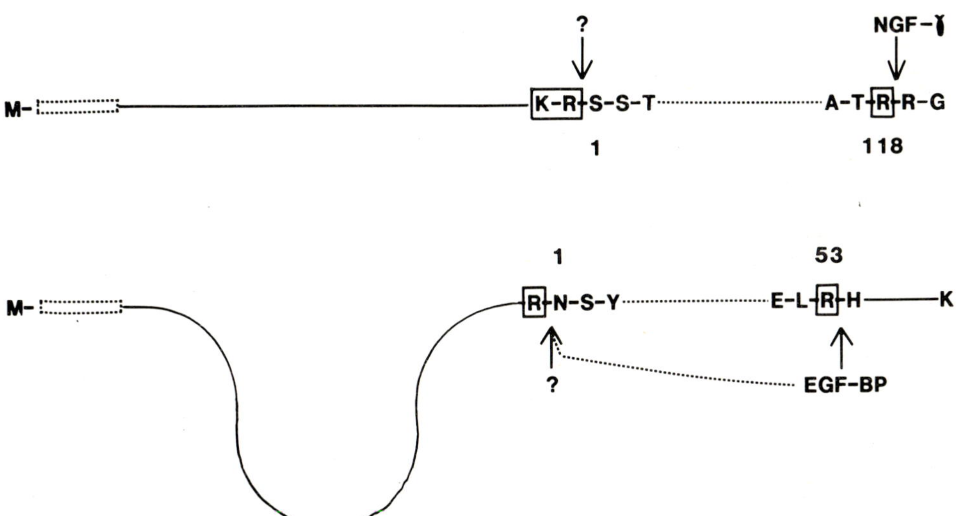

Figure 1. Schematic representation of the precursor structures of mouse nerve growth factor (NGF) (upper) and epidermal growth factor (EGF) (lower). Proteolytic events required to produce the mature hormone in each case are indicated by *solid arrows*. Possible involvements of NGF-γ and EGF-binding protein in these events are indicated. The *dotted box* in each case represents the signal peptide and solid boxed residues represent putative primary recognition sites for the processing enzymes. One letter code for amino acids used; A, alanine; E, glutamic acid; G, glycine; H, histidine; K, lysine; L, leucine; M, methionine; N, asparagine; R, arginine; S, serine; T, threonine; and Y, tyrosine.

12

pancreatic kallikrein. As a result, they have been termed glandular kallikreins. Several identifications of EGF-BP have been reported, the most detailed of which suggested EGF-BP was composed of two proteins (Anundi et al., 1982). Partial amino acid sequences were determined as well as a full length cDNA sequence of one (termed EGF-BP "B") (Lundgren et al., 1984). However, the identification of yet another sequence (Silverman, 1977; Isackson et al., 1987) prompted a reanalysis of this data, which revealed the presence of three unique sequences (Blaber et al., 1987) rather than the two original found. A full length cDNA clone was obtained for this new protein (Blaber et al., 1987) with a sequence distinct from any previous reports. Comparing this sequence as well as the other partial and full sequences proposed for EGF-BP with the genomic structures of the glandular kallikrein family allowed identification of all three genes (mGK-9, mGK-13, and mGK-22) (Drinkwater et al., 1987) found in the preparation of Anundi et al. (1982). Only the protein corresponding to mGK-9, identified by Blaber et al. (1987), has been shown to bind EGF and thus appears to be the principal EGF-BP in this gland.

The three subunits associated with NGF and EGF in the submandibular gland are initially expressed as single chain precursors and each is subsequently cleaved by enzyme(s) unknown (Fig. 2). Following signal peptidase removal of the leader peptide, NGF-γ and EGF-BP are activated by removal of an amino terminal heptapeptide; a similar cleavage does not occur in NGF-α, presumably as the result of interfering mutations (Isackson et al., 1984). Two internal breaks are found in the EGF-BP polypeptide chain and in about half of the molecules in NGF-γ preparations (Thomas et al., 1981); the remaining γ-subunits contain one break, as does NGF-α. Interestingly, in the preparation of EGF-BP described by Anundi et al. (1982), which contains three sequences, the polypeptides contain 0, 1 and 2 internal cleavages, a feature that was essential to establishing the nature of the mixture. The importance of these hydrolyses to function has not been established.

Although the catalytic properties of NGF-γ and EGF-BP are very similar with small synthetic substrates their specificity for interaction with their respective growth factors is apparently highly selective (Server and Shooter, 1976). The binding site for the formation of these complexes is in each case apparently provided by the carboxyl terminal arginine residue of NGF-β and EGF, since derivatives devoid of these residues fail to bind the enzymes. Although direct evidence is lacking, these findings suggest that the kallikreins (EGF-BP and NGF-γ) first bind to the precursor structures, effect the requisite cleavages and then remain associated to the mature hormones as enzyme-product complexes.

Owing to the similarity of the primary structures of EGF-BP and NGF-γ (shown in Fig. 3), only a limited number of differences in these two proteases underlies the specificity of subunit recognition. To identify these residues, molecular models were constructed using the coordinates obtained by X-ray diffraction for bovine trypsin (Blaber M, Blevins RA, Thomas KA, Isackson PJ and Bradshaw RA, manuscript submitted). Into each resulting structure, the peptide corresponding to the last four residues of the mature sequence of each hormone was inserted with the arginine residue placed in the P'-1 site and its α-carboxyl group appropriately juxtaposed to the active center serine. Particular attention was focused on the possible interaction of the glutamic acid residue, the anti-penultimate residue in the carboxyl terminal sequence of EGF, and its possible interaction with a unique, basic residue in the EGF-BP structure. Lysine 215, which is replaced by methionine in the NGF-γ sequence, is found in this vicinity in the model but not close enough to form a stable salt linkage. These findings, supported by kinetic data obtained for variety of tripeptide anilide substrates (Blaber M and Bradshaw RA, unpublished observations), suggest that a selectivity of the interaction of the two glandular kallikreins with their respective mature hormone subunits extends to contacts beyond the active site region.

Nerve Growth Factor in the Guinea Pig Prostate

A second major source of both NGF and EGF, first identified by Harper and

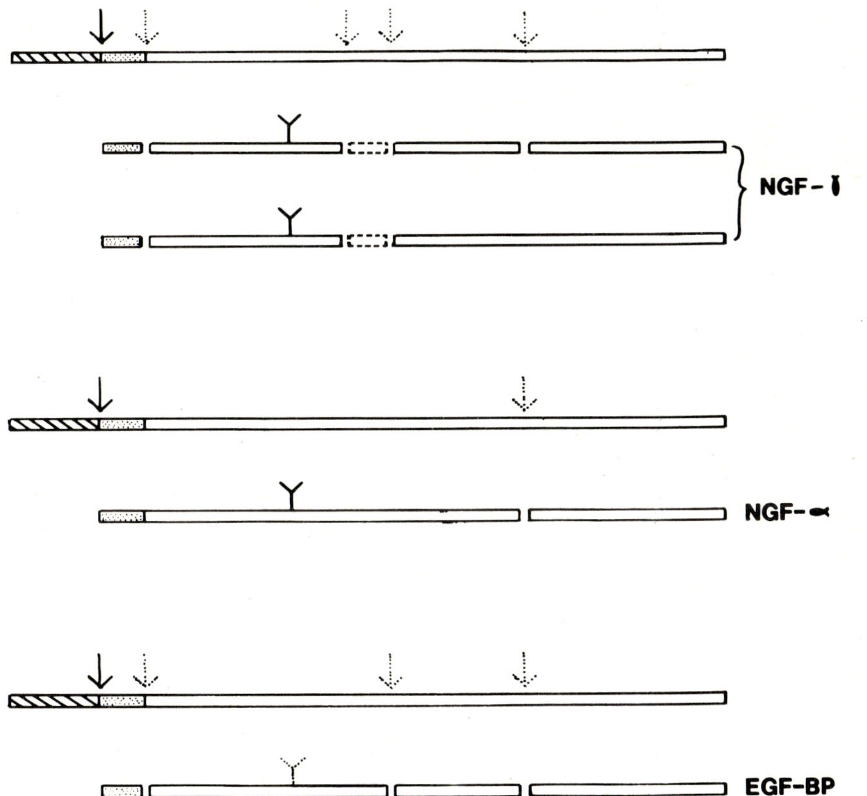

Figure 2. Schematic representation of the precursor and mature forms of the α- and γ-subunits of nerve growth factor and epidermal growth factor binding protein. In each grouping, the top bar (no breaks) represents the prepro structure of each protein. The lower bar(s) of each grouping (with breaks) represents the major mature form(s) derived by various proteolytic events. Cross hatched bars represent signal peptides and stipled bars, pro segments. Sites of signal peptidase activity are indicated by solid arrows; other proteolytic events are indicated by broken arrows. Identified (or putative) carbohydrate sites are indicated by solid or broken Y's respectively.

colleagues (Harper et al., 1979; Harper and Thoenen, 1980a; 1980b), is the prostate gland of several higher vertebrates. The mature forms of each factor, obtained from the corresponding guinea pig tissue, indicate close similarity in both size and primary

```
                                           10                                      20
EGF-BP: I - V - G - G - F - K - C - E - K - N - S - Q - P - W - H - V - A - V - Y - R -
NGF-γ:

                                           30                                      40
EGF-BP: Y - N - E - Y - I - C - G - G - V - L - L - D - A - N - W - V - L - T - A - A -
NGF-γ:  - T -   - Q -       - L -                       - P -

                                           50                                      60
EGF-BP: H - C - Y - Y - E - E - N - K - V - S - L - G - K - N - N - L - Y - E - E - E -
NGF-γ:          - D - D - N - Y -           - W -                       - F - K - D -

                                           70                                      80
EGF-BP: P - S - A - Q - H - R - L - V - S - K - S - F - L - H - P - G - Y - N - R - S -
NGF-γ:                          - F -       - A - I - P -               - F -   - M -

                                           90                                     100
EGF-BP: L - H - R - N - H - I - R - H - P - E - Y - D - Y - S - N - D - L - M - L - L -
NGF-γ:      - M -   - K -           - F - L -

                                          110                                     120
EGF-BP: R - L - S - K - P - A - D - I - T - D - V - V - K - P - I - A - L - P - T - E -
NGF-γ:                                    - T -                   - T -

                                          130                                     140
EGF-BP: E - P - K - L - G - S - T - C - L - A - S - G - W - G - S - T - T - P - F - K -
NGF-γ:                                                        - I -           - T -

                                          150                                     160
EGF-BP: F - Q - N - A - K - D - L - Q - C - V - N - L - K - L - L - P - N - E - D - C -
NGF-γ:      - F - T - D -           - Y -

                                          170                                     180
EGF-BP: G - K - A - H - I - E - K - V - T - D - V - M - L - C - A - G - E - T - D - G -
NGF-γ:  A -                                 - A -                       - M -

                                          190                                     200
EGF-BP: G - K - D - T - C - K - G - D - S - G - G - P - L - I - C - D - G - V - L - Q -
NGF-γ:

                                          210                                     220
EGF-BP: G - I - T - S - W - G - F - T - P - C - G - E - P - K - K - P - G - V - Y - T -
NGF-γ:                          - H -                       - D - M -

                                          230                         237
EGF-BP: K - L - I - K - F - T - S - W - I - K - D - T - M - A - K - N - L
NGF-γ:          - N -                                                   - P
```

Figure 3. Comparison of the amino acid sequences of epidermal growth factor binding protein (EGF-BP) and the γ-subunit of nerve growth factor (NGF-γ). Residues for NGF-γ not listed are identical to those found in EGF-BP. One letter abbreviations: A, alanine; C, half-cystine; D, aspartic acid; E, glutamic acid; F, phenylalanine; G, glycine; H, histidine; I, isoleucine; K, lysine; L, leucine; M, methionine; N, asparagine; P, proline; Q, glutamine; R, arginine; S, serine; T, threonine; V, valine; W, tryptophan; Y, tyrosine. Sequence data taken from Thomas et al. (1981) and Ullrich et al. (1984) (NGF-γ) and Blaber et al. (1987) (EGF-BP).

sequence with the mouse proteins (Rubin and Bradshaw, 1981; Chapman et al., 1981; Rubin, 1983). Interestingly, the NGF and EGF of this tissue is present in extracts largely in unassociated forms. Furthermore, these extracts are entirely devoid of benzoyl arginine-p-nitroanilide activity, the substrate commonly used to assay NGF-γ and EGF-BP. Using tosyl arginine methyl ester as substrate, a single arginine peptidase, not associated with either NGF or EGF, was detected (Dunbar and Bradshaw, 1985), which was ultimately shown to be due to a kallikrein-like enzyme, as judged by its amino acid sequence (Dunbar and Bradshaw, 1987). Although distinctly similar to NGF-γ and EGF-BP, it does possess some unique features, including two sites of glycosylation and a lack of internal cleavages. At present there is no evidence linking this enzyme to processing of precursors for either β-NGF or EGF. In view of the fact that at least guinea pig prostate NGF is elaborated initially in a precursor form, as has been characterized for the mouse protein (Edwards et al., 1986), this would suggest that an enzyme other than NGF-γ catalyzes the conversion of precursor to mature β-NGF in this tissue. The relationship of these activities to potential counterparts in the submaxillary gland is unknown.

Some of the β-NGF activity of the guinea pig prostate is found in a high molecular weight complex, albeit at a somewhat lower molecular weight than the corresponding 7S complex of the mouse submaxillary gland (Schwarz M, Dunbar J, Rubin JS and Bradshaw RA, unpublished results). The NGF activity present in this complex is recognized by antisera to mouse β-NGF and is reduced on SDS polyacrylamide gel electrophoresis to the same molecular weight as the mouse β-NGF subunit. The nature of the material complexed with the β-NGF subunit in this form of the hormone is not known. It does not contain catalytic activity reminiscent of kallikreins, nor are there present polypeptide chains of a molecular weight expected for either α- or γ-type molecules (Schwarz M, Isackson PJ and Bradshaw RA, unpublished results). Interestingly, two other peaks of NGF-like activity, as identified using a PC-12 cell neurite outgrowth assay, are present in guinea pig prostate extracts. These activities, which are not cross-reactive with the same antisera, can be distinguished from the material that is cross-reactive by their position on a gel filtration column. NGF has been partially characterized in bovine seminal plasma (Harper et al., 1982); in seminal vesicle tissue of the guinea pig, only one active entity has been identified which does not crossreact with mouse β-NGF antisera. Whether this activity is the same as one of the two components not cross-reactive with mouse β-NGF antisera in the prostate extract remains to be determined. The molecular characteristics of these neurotrophic factors are presently under investigation.

FUNCTION

Epidermal Growth Factor in the Central Nervous System

Epidermal growth factor, which was first identified in mouse submaxillary gland extracts as a molecule able to induce premature eyelid opening and incisor eruption (Cohen, 1962) has been characterized functionally primarily as a mitogen for epithelial tissue (Haigler, 1983) and as a gastrointestinal hormone (Gregory, 1980). Recently,

Fallon et al. (1984) identified immuno crossreactive material in the brain of neonatal rats that suggested a possible role for EGF (or an EGF-like peptide) in the CNS. This material had a narrow distribution being located only in the pallidal region. These findings were consistent with reports that small but detectable levels of mRNA for EGF were present in the brain (Rall et al., 1985).

A strong indication of a physiological role for EGF in the CNS was provided by observations that striatal neurons of neonatal rats when cultured in the presence of EGF responded dramatically in terms of increased survival and process outgrowth relative to untreated controls (Morrison et al., 1987). The same cultures were unresponsive to a variety of other mitogenic substances including thrombin and platelet-derived growth factor, although they did respond to bFGF. This is in keeping with previous observations that bFGF can also stimulate hippocampal and cortical neurons in a similar fashion (Walicke et al., 1986; Morrison et al., 1986).

The effect of EGF can be observed over a period of two weeks and withdrawal of the hormone during that period results in the ultimate death of the surviving neurons. Dose response curves suggest that a half optimal dose of the hormone is 1 nanogram. This is effectively the same concentration required for mitogenic responses to EGF in appropriately responding cells. It was also observed that transforming growth factor α (TGF-α), an analog of EGF with limited similarity in amino acid sequence (Marquardt et al., 1983), can substitute for EGF in these responses. This is also in keeping with other observations that TGF-α can act as a mitogen for EGF responsive cells by cross-reaction with the EGF receptor (Massague, 1983; Tam et al., 1984). These results imply, but do not establish, that the receptors for EGF on the responsive neurons in these preparations are similar or identical to those characteristic of mitogenically responsive cells.

NGF and bFGF Responses with Pheochromocytoma (PC-12) Cells

The pheochromocytoma cell line (PC-12), originally established by Greene and Tischler (1976) has proven to be an important paradigm for studying growth factor mechanism of action and the molecular basis of differentiation. That cell line responds to exposure to β-NGF by attaching to substratum and extending neuronal-like processes that are entirely reminiscent of sympathetic neurons. A variety of additional morphological, physiological and biochemical changes accompany this response (Greene and Tischler, 1982). Interestingly, withdrawal of a hormone results in the reversal of the process. Similar responses have been induced by dibutyryl cyclic AMP (Halegoua and Patrick, 1980), the viral oncogenes *src* (Alema et al., 1985) and *ras* (Bar-Sagi and Feramisco, 1985), and bFGF (Togari et al., 1983; Rydel and Greene, 1987; Neufeld et al., 1987; Eveleth DD and Bradshaw RA, unpublished observations). PC-12 cells also recognize and bind EGF but the biological response induced is basically the opposite of that induced by NGF (Huff and Guroff, 1979).

The NGF response is initiated by formation of complexes at the cell surface with high affinity receptors. PC-12 cells like other responsive neurons also contain low affinity receptors for NGF, the principal component of which has been recently cloned and sequenced (Radeke et al., 1987). The cDNA for a similar structure from human melanoma cells has also been identified and sequenced (Chao et al., 1986). The relationship of this entity to the high affinity receptor in either PC-12 cells or other responsive tissues remains to be elucidated. These two entities may be entirely different in structure or they may be related by the association of an additional specifying agent (Yankner and Shooter, 1982; Kouchalakos and Bradshaw, 1986).

To address this issue, we have examined the mutant cell line of the parent PC-12 clone, designated nnr5 for NGF nonresponsive (Green et al., 1986). These cells were originally described as being defective in the high-affinity NGF receptor, thus causing the lack of response to this hormone; they remain responsive to cAMP. However, these cells were also found to be unresponsive to bFGF (Eveleth DD, Schwarz M and Bradshaw RA, unpublished observations). These observations suggest that the defect may lay elsewhere, perhaps in the pathway common to the NGF and bFGF stimulation. Consistent with that idea is the fact that these cells are competent to internalize NGF, as judged by protection of bound I^{125}-NGF to acid washes, but are unable to degrade this sequestered hormone by the usual lysosomal route. Thus, these findings suggest that nnr5 cells may be defective in the receptor-mediated endocytosis pathway that governs NGF and FGF responses. Since these cells are competent to internalize and degrade EGF, the defect is not found in that portion of the endocytosis pathway utilized by this ligand.

Clearly, receptor-mediated endocytosis, a common feature in growth factor responses involving both hypertrophic and hyperplastic stimulation (James and Bradshaw, 1984), may play an essential role in the transmembrane signalling process.

The bFGF receptor of PC-12 cells appear similar in several of its characteristics to that found in other mitotically responsive cell types (Neufeld and Gospodarowicz, 1986; Olwin and Hauschka, 1986). Covalent crosslinking with I^{125} bFGF reveals a single band on SDS cell electrophoresis of Mr 160,000 consistent with a molecular mass of the receptor entity of 145 kDa. The affinity of this receptor for bFGF is comparable with that observed in other cell types as reflected in similar dose-response curves. These findings suggest that the receptor for FGF on PC-12 cells will be similar, if not identical, to that found in cells which are induced to divide under the influence of this hormone. Taken with the observations of EGF stimulation of central nervous system neurons to undergo hypertrophic but not hyperplastic responses, there is a recognizable pattern that suggests that receptors for various ligands may be involved in either hyperplastic or hypertrophic responses and that it is neither the character of the ligand nor the receptor (or any of its inherent properties) that are involved in this decision, but rather the internal pathways with which they are connected. Thus it is arbitrary and almost certainly inappropriate to limit growth factors to those substances with mitogenic activity since this distinction appears to be related to the state of differentiation of the target cells rather than any inherent property of the factors themselves.

SUMMARY

Although there has been casual identification of a considerable number of neurotrophic factors as judged by variety of assays measuring neuronal survival, process extension or modulation of phenotypic expression, very few of these have been purifed to homogeneity and subsequently characterized with respect to molecular properties. Although the problems in isolation of these molecules can be readily traced to instability and low concentrations, difficulties with reproducible assays have also contributed to the problem. Interestingly, these failures have helped to maintain and perhaps proliferate the concept that there is a wide variety of neurotrophic factors that influence both the peripheral and the central nervous systems both during development and in their respective mature states.

As illustrated by the findings presented in this article, the number of neurotrophic factors may be somewhat more proscribed. Clearly the identification of EGF and bFGF as important neurotrophic factors for the CNS with potentially a broad spectrum of neuronal targets suggests that the specificity anticipated in the maintenance of CNS may not come so much from the numbers of different neurotrophic factors as their combinatorial effects on responsive neurons. That is to say, neurotrophic factors may in fact be largely made up of substances which also function as mitogens (or in other capacities) elsewhere in the organism. Improved understanding of the biosynthesis of these entities, including the identification of their sites of synthesis and the manner in which the mature forms are elaborated and secreted, will aid in our appreciation of their full range of physiological functions.

ACKNOWLEDGMENTS

Studies arising from the authors laboratories were supported by research grants from the U.S.P.H.S. (DK32465, NS19964, NS19319 and program project grant AG00538) and the American Cancer Society (BC273). M.B. is supported by a U.S.P.H.S. Predoctoral Training Grant, GM07134, K.C. is a fellow of the Hereditary Disease Foundation, D.D.E. is a fellow of the Bank of America-Gianini Foundation, R.S.M. was supported by U.S.P.H.S. Training Grant CA0905A, and M.S. was a U.S.P.H.S. Post-doctoral Fellow, NS07803. The authors would like to thank Marja Uskali for the expert assistance in the preparation of the manuscript.

REFERENCES

Alema S, Casalbore P, Agostini E, Tato F (1985) Differentiation of PC12 phaeochromocytoma cells induced by v-*src* oncogene. Nature 316:557-559.

Anundi H, Ronne H, Peterson PA, Rask L (1982) Partial amino-acid sequence of the epidermal growth-factor-binding protein. Eur J Biochem 129:365-371.

Barde Y-A, Edgar D, Thoenen H (1983) New neurotrophic factors. Ann Rev Physiol 45:601-612.

Bar-Sagi D, Feramisco J (1985) Microinjection of the *ras* oncogene protein into PC12 cells induced morphological differentiation. Cell 42:841-848.

Berg DK (1984) New neuronal growth factors. Ann Rev Neurosci 7:149-170.

Berger B, Wise C, Stein L (1973) Nerve growth factor: enhanced recovery of feeding after hypothalamic damage. Science 180:506-508.

Blaber M, Isackson PJ, Bradshaw RA (1987) A complete cDNA sequence for the major epidermal growth factor binding protein in the male mouse submandibular gland. Biochemistry 26 (21):6742-6749.

Chao MW, Bothwell MA, Ross AH, Koprowski H, Lonahan A, Buck CR, Sehgal A (1986) Gene transfer and molecular cloning of the human NGF receptor. Science 232:418-421.

Chapman B, Banks CB, Vernon CA, Walker JM (1982) Isolation and characterization of nerve growth factor from the prostate gland of the guinea-pig. Eur J Biochem 115:347-351.

Cohen S (1962) Isolation of a mouse submaxillary gland protein accelerating incisor eruption and eyelid opening in the newborn animal. J Biol Chem 237:1555-1562.

Davies AM, Bandtlow C, Heumann R, Korsching S, Rohrer H, Thoenen H (1987) Timing and site of nerve growth factor synthesis in developing skin in relation to innervation and expression of the receptor. Nature 326:353-358.

Drinkwater CC, Evans BA, Richards RI (1987) Mouse glandular kallikrein genes: identification and characterization of the genes encoding the epidermal growth factor-binding proteins. Biochemistry 26 (21):6750-6756.

Dunbar J, Bradshaw RA (1985) Nerve growth factor biosynthesis: Isolation and characterization of a guinea pig prostate kallikrein. J Cell Biochem 29:309-319.

Dunbar J, Bradshaw RA (1987) Amino acid sequence of guinea pig prostate kallikrein. Biochemistry 26:3471-3478.

Edwards RH, Selby MJ, Rutter WJ (1986) Differential RNA splicing predicts two distinct nerve growth factor precursors. Nature 319: 784-787.

Evans BA, Drinkwater CC, Richards RI (1987) Mouse glandular kallikrein genes - structure and partial sequence analysis of the kallikrein gene locus. J Biol Chem 262:8027-8034.

Fallon JH, Seroogy KO, Loughlin SE, Morrison RS, Bradshaw RA, Knauer DJ, Cunningham DD (1984) Epidermal growth factor - immunoreactive material in the central nervous system: location and development. Science 224:1107-1109.

Fischer W, Wictorin K, Bjorklund A, Williams LR, Varon S, Gage FH (1987) Amelioration of cholinergic neuron atrophy and spatial memory impairment in aged rats by nerve growth factor. Nature: 329:65-68.

Gnahn H, Hefti F, Heumann R, Schwab ME, Thoenen H (1983) NGF-mediated increase of choline acetyltransferase (CHAT) in the neonatal rat forebrain: Evidence for a physiological role of NGF in the brain? Dev Brain Res 9:45-52.

Gospadarowicz D, Cheng K, Lui G-M, Baird A, Bohlen P (1984) Isolation of brain fibroblast growth factor by heparin-Sepharose affinity chromatography: Identity with pituitary fibroblast growth factor. Proc Natl Acad Sci USA 81:6963-6967.

Gray A, Dull TJ, Ullrich A (1983) Nucleotide sequence of epidermal growth factor cDNA predicts a 128,000-molecular weight protein precursor. Nature 303:722-725.

Green E, Rydel SH, Connolly JL, Greene LA (1986) PC12 cell mutant that possess low but not high affinity nerve growth factor receptors neither respond to nor internalize nerve growth factor. J Cell Biol 102:830-843.

Greene LA, Shooter EM (1980) The nerve growth factor: biochemistry, synthesis, and mechanism of action. Ann Rev Neurosci 3:353-402.

Greene LA, Shooter EM, Varon S (1968) Enzymatic activities of mouse nerve growth factor and its subunits. Proc Natl Acad Sci USA 60:1383-1388.

Greene LA, Tischler AS (1976) Establishment of a noradrenergic clonal cell line of rat pheochromocytoma cells which respond to nerve growth factor. Proc Natl Acad Sci USA 73:2424-2428.

Greene LA, Tischler AS (1982) PC12 pheochromocytoma cultures in neurobiological research. Adv Cell Neurobiol 3: 373-414.

Gregory H (1980) Urogastrone: Isolation, structure and basic functions. In: George B. Jerzy Glass (ed): Gastrointestinal hormones. Raven Press, N.Y., pp. 397-409.

Haigler HT (1983) Epidermal Growth Factor: Cellular binding and consequences. In: Guroff G (ed): Growth and Maturation Factors. John Wiley & Sons, NY, pp. 117-154.

20

Halegoua S, Patrick J (1980) Nerve growth factor mediates phosphorylation of specific proteins. Cell 22:571-581.

Harper GP, Barde YA, Burnstock G, Carstairs JR, Dennison ME, Suda K, Vernon CA (1979) Guinea pig prostate is a rich source of nerve growth factor. Nature 279:160-162.

Harper GP, Glanville RW, Thoenen H (1982) The purification of nerve growth factor from bovine seminal plasma. J Biol Chem 257:9541-9548.

Harper GP, Thoenen H (1980a) The distribution of nerve growth factor in the male sex organs of mammals. J Neurochem 34:893-903.

Harper GP, Thoenen H (1980b) Nerve growth factor: Biological significance, measurement, and distribution. J Neurochem 34:5-15.

Hart T, Chamais N, Moore RY, Stein D (1978) Effects of nerve growth factor on behavioral recovery following caudate nucleus lesions in rats. Brain Res Bull 3:245-250.

Hefti F, Dravid A, Hartikka J (1984) Chronic intraventricular injections of nerve growth factor elevate hippocampal choline acetyltransferase activity in adult rats with partial septo-hippocampal lesions. Brain Res 293:305-311.

Hefti F, Hartikka J, Eckenstein J, Gnahn F, Heumann R, Schwab M (1985) Nerve growth factor increases choline acetyltransferase but not survival or fiber outgrowth of cultured septal cholinergic neurons. Neurosci 14:55-68.

Honegger P, Lenoir D (1983) Nerve growth factor (NGF) stimulation of cholinergic telencephalic neurons in aggregating cell cultures. Dev Brain Res 3:229-238.

Huff KR, Guroff G (1979) Nerve growth factor induced reduction in epidermal growth factor responsiveness and epidermal growth factor receptors in PC12 cells: an aspect of cell differentiation. Biochem Biophys Res Commun 89:175-180.

Isackson PJ, Bradshaw RA (1984) The α-subunit of mouse 7S nerve growth factor is an inactive serine protease. J Biol Chem 259:5380-5383.

Isackson PJ, Silverman RE, Blaber M, Server AC, Nichols RA, Shooter EM, Bradshaw RA (1987) Epidermal growth factor binding protein: Identification of a different protein. Biochem 26:2082-2085.

Isackson PJ, Ullrich A, Bradshaw RA (1984) Mouse 7S nerve growth factor: Complete sequence of a cDNA coding for the α-subunit precursor and its relationship to serine proteases. Biochem 23:5997-6002.

James R, Bradshaw RA (1984) Polypeptide growth factors. Ann Rev Biochem 53:259-292.

Kouchalakos R, Bradshaw RA (1986) Nerve growth factor receptor from rabbit sympathetic ganglia membranes: relationship between subforms. J Biol Chem 261:16054-16059.

Levi-Montalcini R (1987) The nerve growth factor 35 years later. Science 237:1154-1162.

Lewis M, Brown M, Brownstein M, Hart T, Stein DG (1979) Nerve growth factor: effects on D-amphetamine-induced activity and brain monoamines. Brain Res 176:297-310.

Lobb R, Sasse J, Sullivan R, Shing Y, D'Amore P, Jacobs J, Klagsburn M (1986) Purification and characterization of heparin-binding endothelial cell growth factors. J Biol Chem 261:1924-1928.

Lundgren S, Ronne H, Rask L, Peterson PA (1984) Sequence of an epidermal growth factor-binding protein. J Biol Chem 259:7780-7784.

Marquardt H, Hunkapiller MW, Hood LE, Twardzik DR, de Larco JE, Stephenson JR, Todaro GJ (1983) Transforming growth factors produced by retrovirus-transformed rodent fibroblasts and human melanoma cells: amino acid sequence homology with epidermal growth factor. Proc Natl Acad Sci USA 80:4684-4688.

Mason AJ, Evans BA, Cox DR, Shine J, Richards RI (1983) Structure of mouse kallikrein gene family suggests a role in specific processing of biologically active peptides. Nature 303:300-307.

Massague J (1983) Epidermal growth factor-like transforming growth factor II. Interactions with epidermal growth factor receptors in human placenta membranes and A431 cells. J Biol Chem 258: 13614-13620.

Mobley WC, Rutkowski JL, Tennekoon GI, Buchanan K, Johnston MV (1985) Choline acetyltransferase activity in striatum of neonatal rats increased by nerve growth factor. Science 229:284-287.

Morrison RS, Kornblum HI, Leslie FM, Bradshaw RA (1987) Trophic stimulation of subcortical neurons of neonatal rat brain by epidermal growth factor. Science 238 (4823):72-75.

Morrison RS, Sharma A, de Vellis J, Bradshaw RA (1986) Basic fibroblast growth factor supports the survival of cerebral cortical neurons in primary culture. Proc Natl Acad Sci USA 83:7537-7541.

Neufeld G, Gospadarowicz D (1986) Basic and acidic fibroblast growth factors interact with the same cell surface receptors. J Biol Chem 261:5631-5637.

Neufeld G, Gospadarowicz D, Dodge L, Fuji DK (1987) Heparin modulation of the neurotrophic effects of acidic and basic fibroblast growth factors and nerve growth factor on PC12 cells. J Cell Physiol 131:131-140.

Olwin BB, Hauschka SD (1986) Identification of the fibroblast growth factor receptor of Swiss 3T3 cells and mouse skeletal muscle myoblasts. Biochem 25:3487-3492.

Probstmeier R, Schachner M (1986) Epidermal growth factor is not detectable in developing an adult brain by a sensitive double-site enzyme immunoassay. Neurosci Lett 63:290-294.

Radeke MJ, Misko TP, Hsu C, Herzenberg LA, Shooter EM (1987) Gene transfer and molecular cloning of the rat nerve growth factor receptor. Nature 325:593-597.

Rall LB, Scott J, Bell GI, Crawford RJ, Penschow JD, Niall HD, Coghlan JP (1985) Mouse prepro-epidermal growth factor synthesis by the kidney and other tissues. Nature 313:228-231.

Ronne H, Anundi H, Rask L, Peterson PA (1984) 7S nerve growth factor α and γ subunits are closely related proteins. Biochem 23:1229-1234.

Rubin JS (1983) Purification and characterization of three polypeptide growth factors from mammalian sources. Ph.D. Thesis, Washington Univ, St. Louis, MO.

Rubin JS, Bradshaw RA (1981) Isolation and partial amino acid sequence analysis of nerve growth factor from the guinea pig prostate. J Neurosci Res 6:451-464.

Rush RA (1984) Immunohistochemical localization of endogenous nerve growth factor. Nature 312:364-367.

Rydel ER, Greene LA (1987) Acidic and basic fibroblast growth factors promote stable neurite outgrowth and neuronal differentiation in cultures of PC12 cells. J Neurosci, in press.

Scott J, Selby M, Urdea M, Quiroga M, Bell GI, Rutter WJ (1983a) Isolation and nucleotide sequence of a cDNA encoding the precursor of mouse nerve growth factor. Nature 302:538-540.

Scott J, Urdea M, Quiroga M, Sanchez-Pescador R, Fong N, Selby N, Rutter WJ, Bell GI (1983b) Structure of a mouse submaxillary messenger RNA encoding epidermal growth factor and seven related proteins. Science 221:236-240.

Server AC, Shooter EM (1976) Comparison of the arginine esteropeptidases associated with the nerve and epidermal growth factors. J Biol Chem 251:165-173.

Silverman RE (1977) Interactions within the mouse nerve growth factor complex. Ph.D. Thesis, Washington Univ, St. Louis, MO.

Tam JP, Marquardt H, Rosberger D, Heath NY, Todaro GJ (1984) Synthesis of biologically active rat transforming growth factor I. Nature 309:376-378.

Taylor JM, Mitchell WM, Cohen S (1974) Characterization of the binding protein for epidermal growth factor. J Biol Chem 249:2188-2194.

Thomas KA, Baglan NC, Bradshaw RA (1981) The amino acid sequence of the γ-subunit of mouse submaxillary gland 7S nerve growth factor. J Biol Chem 256:9156-9166.

Togari A, Baker D, Dickens G, Guroff G (1983) The neurite-promoting effect of fibroblast growth factor on PC12 cells. J Neurosci 5:307-316.

Ullrich A, Gray A, Berman C, Dull TJ (1983) Human β-nerve growth factor gene sequence highly homologous to that of mouse. Nature 303:821-825.

Ullrich A, Gray A, Wood W, Hayflick J, Seeberg PH (1984) Isolation of a cDNA clone coding for the γ-subunit of mouse nerve growth factor using a high-stringency selection procedure. DNA 3:387-392.

Walicke P, Cowan WM, Veno N, Baird A, Guillemin R (1986) Fibroblast growth factor promotes survival of dissociated hippocampal neurons and enhances neurite extension. Proc Natl Acad Sci USA 83:3012-3016.

Yankner BA, Shooter EM (1982) The biology and mechanism of action of nerve growth factor. Ann Rev Biochem 51:845-868.

Neuronal Plasticity and Trophic Factors
G. Biggio, P.F. Spano, G. Toffano, S.H. Appel, G.L. Gessa (eds.)
Fidia Research Series, Symposia in Neuroscience VII
Liviana Press, Padova © 1988

LEVELS OF NERVE GROWTH FACTOR AND ITS mRNA DURING DEVELOPMENT AND REGENERATION OF THE PERIPHERAL NERVOUS SYSTEM

Sigrun Korsching, Rolf Heumann, Alun M. Davies and Hans Thoenen

Max-Planck-Institut für Psychiatrie, Abteilung für Neurochemie,
D-8033 Martinsried, FRG

INTRODUCTION

Nerve growth factor (NGF) is essential for the survival of sympathetic and sensory neurons during early periods of their development and it enhances differentiation of these and some central cholinergic neurons during later periods (Levi-Montalcini and Angeletti 1968; Thoenen and Barde 1980; Korsching, 1986). For example, NGF increases tyrosine hydroxylase activity in sympathetic neurons and substance P content in a subpopulation of sensory neurons. Deprival of endogenous NGF by injection of specific antibodies leads to the death of these neurons, thereby showing that NGF is indeed a physiological factor used by and necessary for sympathetic and sensory neurons during development *in vivo* (Thoenen and Barde, 1980). However, the endogenous source of NGF for these neurons has long remained elusive. Several years ago, the only *bona fide* source of NGF in the mouse has been the submandibular gland, whose huge content of NGF had made possible the isolation and characterization of this factor in the first place (Levi-Montalcini and Angeletti, 1968). Although the actual function, if any, of this rich source of NGF remains unknown, it is clear that in this exocrine gland

---

Abbreviations: NGF: nerve growth factor, SCG: superior cervical ganglion, E: embryonic day.
Present addresses: Sigrun Korsching: California Institute of Technology, Division of Biology 216-76, Pasadena, CA 91125, USA; Alun M. Davies: St. George's Hospital Medical School, Dept. of Anatomy, London SW17 ORE, UK.

NGF is secreted into the saliva so that it does not gain access to the innervating neurons (Levi-Montalcini and Angeletti, 1968).

Despite the absence of information about the physiologically relevant sites of NGF production, three sets of observations were taken to suggest a model for the function of NGF in the organism:

1. labeled NGF injected in the target regions of sympathetic, sensory and magnocellular cholinergic neurons is subject to specific retrograde transport within the axons of these neurons;

2. interruption of retrograde axonal transport in sympathetic neurons mimics the effects of withdrawal of NGF by antibodies; and

3. these neurons can be rescued by addition of exogenous NGF (Thoenen and Barde, 1980; Korsching, 1986).

These observations suggested the following model: NGF is synthesized in target organs of the sympathetic and sensory nervous system and secreted, followed by a specific, receptor-mediated uptake into endocytotic vesicles of these neurons. NGF is then delivered to the neuronal soma by retrograde axonal transport, where NGF (or a co-transported second messenger) exerts its effects and finally is degraded in lysosomal vesicles.

We have tested the predictions of this model concerning the synthesis and distribution of NGF. To this end, we developed a specific and quantitative two-site enzyme immunoassay for the determination of NGF (Korsching and Thoenen, 1987) with a detection limit of 50-100 pg NGF/g wet weight. mRNA^{NGF} was determined by quantitative Northern blots using a RNA probe with a detection limit of 5-10 pg mRNA^{NGF}/g wet weight (Heumann and Thoenen, 1986). A short summary of the results for adult tissues is shown in Figure 1. The main features are:

— mRNA^{NGF} and NGF are specifically present in target tissues of sympathetic and a subpopulation of sensory neurons. NGF is not found in rat serum, in other words, it is not an endocrine factor but is locally synthesized in target tissues of NGF-responsive neurons. Synthesis of NGF is roughly correlated with the density of sympathetic innervation the target tissue receives, as graphically represented in Figure 1. Similar results for the distribution of mRNA^{NGF} have been obtained by Shelton and Reichardt (1984).

— Sympathetic ganglia and sciatic nerve contain high levels of NGF but essentially no mRNA^{NGF}; e.g. the ratio of mRNA^{NGF} to NGF is about 30-fold lower for sciatic nerve than for sympathetic target organs. This indicates that NGF is not synthesized in nerve or ganglia but merely transported in the axons.

This analysis of steady state levels for NGF meets the expectations for NGF synthesis based on the retrograde trophic messenger model for NGF. We have then investigated the distribution of NGF following interruption of retrograde axonal transport. The mechanical blockade of axonal transport by crushing the sciatic nerve leads to a rapid accumulation of NGF distal to the crush, reaching maximal values 12 h post crush (Fig. 2b), whereas NGF levels decreased well below control levels proximal to the crush. This asymmetric accumulation of NGF is direct evidence of retrograde axonal transport of endogenous NGF and in good accordance with the results of

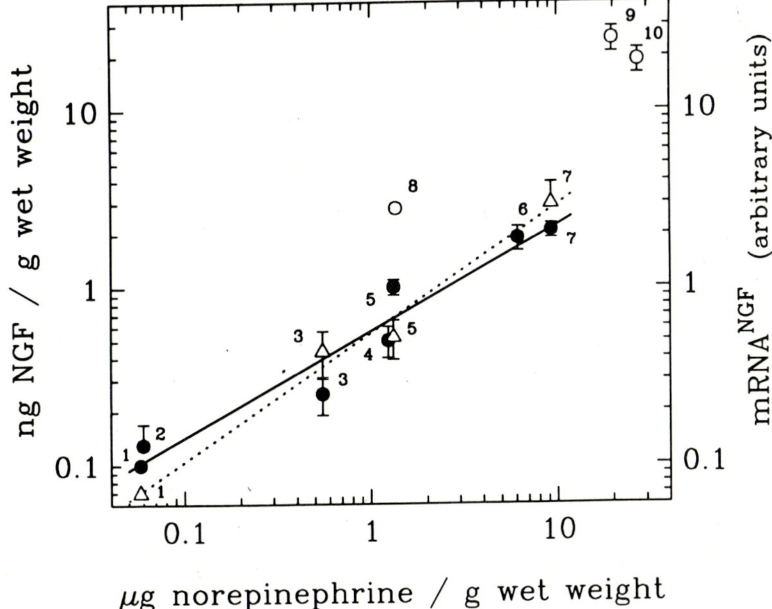

Figure 1. Correlation between NGF or mRNA^{NGF} content and the density of sympathetic innervation as measured by the norepinephrine content. Data are for rat (NGF) and mouse organs (mRNA^{NGF}), respectively. Means $\pm$ SEM are taken from Korsching and Thoenen, 1983a, Korsching, 1984 and Heumann et al., 1984. The norepinephrine content is the mean for all determinations given in Holzbauer and Sharman (1972) for the respective organs. ●-● NGF content of different target organs as function of their norepinephrine content. According to increasing norepinephrine content: 1) skeletal muscle [detection limit], 2) liver, 3) heart ventricle, 4) submandibular gland, 5) heart atrium, 6) iris, 7) vas deferens. ○-○ NGF content of ganglia and nerve as function of NE content: 8) sciatic nerve, 9) SCG, 10) stellate ganglion. △-△ mRNA^{NGF} content of 1) skeletal muscle [detection limit], 3) heart ventricle, 5) heart atrium, 7) vas deferens. Both straight lines are least square fits of the doublelogarithmic plot, – for the NGF content of the target organs, and ... for their mRNA^{NGF} content.

immunohistochemical localization after a sympathetic nerve crush by Palmatier et al. (1984). Interruption of retrograde axonal transport specifically in the sympathetic nervous system has been achieved by injection of 6-OH-dopamine, which in adult animals destroys only sympathetic nerve terminals. A subsequent rapid accumulation of NGF in the sympathetically innervated organs is accompanied by a drastic decrease of NGF levels in the sympathetic ganglia down to less than 5% of control values within 24 h (Fig. 2a, c). Again, this confirms the notion of NGF as a target organ-derived factor. The increase of NGF in the target organs mainly seems to be due to the inhibition of removal by retrograde axonal transport, since the rate of synthesis, as measured by the amount of mRNA^{NGF} present, does not change after sympathetic denervation (Shelton and Reichardt, 1986).

From these data we can conclude that NGF is synthesized in target organs of sympathetic neurons, that these neurons obtain NGF *via* retrograde axonal transport from the organs they innervate and, finally, that the synthesis of NGF in target organs is correlated with their density of sympathetic innervation. Is there a causal relation underlying this correlation? More precisely, might the amount of NGF synthesis in target organs determine the density of sympathetic innervation during development and possibly even serve to attract these fibers to their correct target organs in the first place? This is a tempting hypothesis since it has been shown that NGF can exert chemotactic guidance on both sympathetic and sensory neurons (Gundersen and Barrett, 1979; Levi-Montalcini et al., 1978). To study these questions we have analysed the distribution of NGF and its mRNA during development of the sympathetic and the sensory nervous system.

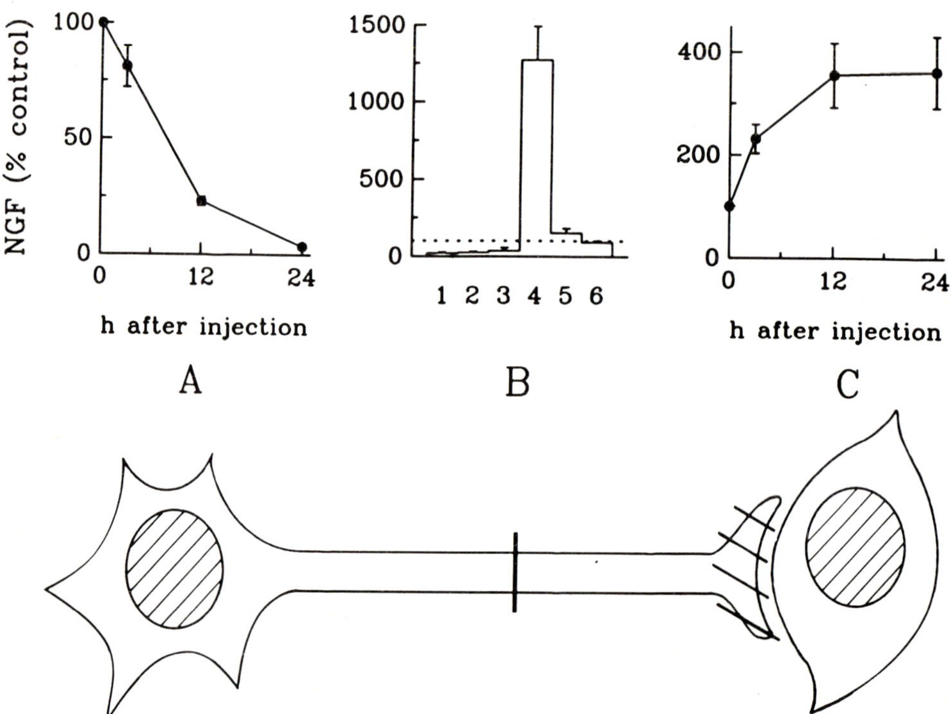

Figure 2. NGF content, expressed as % of control, after systemic (panel A, C) or local (B) blockade of axonal transport. Data are means ± SEM and taken from Korsching and Thoenen 1983b, 1985. The lower panel shows the schematic representation of both experiments, ganglia to the left, nerve in the middle, and innervated organ to the right. A: NGF content of the rat stellate ganglion after a single systemic injection of 6-OH-dopamine. B: NGF content of rat sciatic nerve 12 h after a crush. Numbers 1 to 6 correspond to segments of 2 mm length each, Nr. 1 being the most proximal segment; crush as indicated between segment 3 and 4. C: NGF content of the heart atrium, a target organ of the stellate ganglion, after injection of 6-OH-dopamine.

As model system for sensory neurons we have chosen the trigeminal ganglion of the mouse and its major target area, the whisker pad region. The time course of innervation in this system has been described by Davies and Lumsden (1984). In the target region both mRNA^{NGF} and NGF itself are first detectable at embryonic day (E) 11, which is exactly the time when the first sensory axons reach their target (Fig. 3a,b). The NGF content then rises 21-fold to reach maximal values at E13 and thereafter decreases markedly, although the NGF synthesis, as measured by the amount of mRNA^{NGF} present, is still increasing somewhat. This apparent inconsistency is resolved by analysis of the trigeminal ganglion, where NGF first appears at E12, one day later than in the target region; NGF then increases drastically throughout the period when NGF is decreasing in the whisker pad (Fig. 3b). It seems therefore most likely that the decrease in whisker pad NGF levels after E13 is caused by the increasing magnitude of retrograde axonal transport of NGF to the trigeminal ganglion, leading to the increase in ganglionic NGF levels. As late as E15 and E16, no mRNA for NGF was detectable in the trigeminal ganglion, indicating that in accordance with the above interpretation and in parallel to the situation in the mature nervous system, NGF present in the ganglion is derived from the target organs and does not stem from local synthesis by nonneuronal cells within the ganglion.

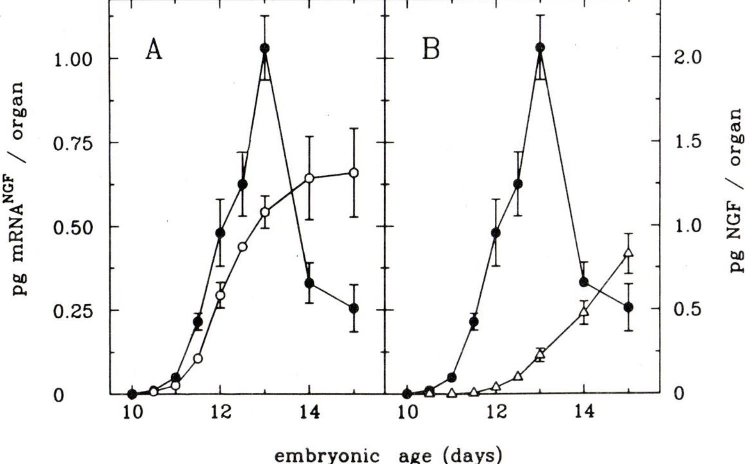

Figure 3. Developmental time course of NGF and mRNA^{NGF} levels in the whisker pad and trigeminal ganglion of the mouse. The time period is embryonic day 10 to 15. Data are means $\pm$ SEM and taken from Davies et al., 1987. The y-axis to the left shows the mRNA^{NGF} content in pg/organ and the y-axis to the right shows the NGF content in pg/organ. Error bars smaller than the symbol size were omitted. NGF levels for E10, E10.5 and mRNA^{NGF} levels for E10 were not significantly different from zero. A: ○–○ mRNA^{NGF} content of the whisker pad, the major target organ of the trigeminal ganglion; ●–● NGF content of the whisker pad. B: △–△ NGF content of the trigeminal ganglion, ●–● for comparison again the NGF content of the whisker pad.

Within the target organ, mRNA^{NGF} levels in the epithelial cell layer are severalfold higher than in the underlying mesodermal layer (Davies et al., 1987). Since the epithelial layer receives much denser sensory innervation than the mesodermal layer, this indicates a correlation of NGF synthesis with the density of sensory innervation.

The absence of detectable NGF in the sensory target organ prior to its innervation argues against the possibility of NGF exerting a chemotactic influence to guide the first innervating neurons towards their correct target. In fact, these neurons lack detectable NGF receptors prior to contact with the target. Explants of E10 trigeminal ganglia begin to express NGF receptors after 1 day in culture (presumably corresponding to E11), as detected by light-microscopic autoradiography after binding of ^{125}I-labeled NGF (Davies et al., 1987). It is noteworthy that both NGF synthesis and expression of NGF receptors begin at the time when the axons first contact the target. However, at least in chicken, NGF synthesis in target organs does not depend on the presence of neural crest or neural tube-derived innervation (Thoenen et al., unpublished observations).

In support of these findings with sensory targets, in the heart ventricle and the submandibular gland, both target organs of sympathetic neurons, NGF is first detectable around the time of initial innervation by sympathetic neurons (embryonic day 12 and 13, respectively). The time course for submandibular gland is shown in Figure 4. After a 14-fold increase in the next three days, NGF levels remain in the ng NGF/g wet weight range for the whole perinatal period, i.e. they remain subsaturating for the whole period of neuronal death. This is to be expected, since addition of exogenous NGF during this time period can prevent the naturally occurring death of sympathetic neurons

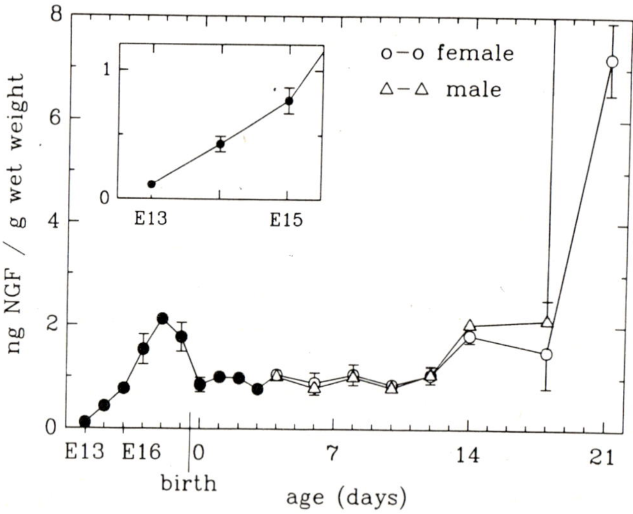

Figure 4. Developmental time course of NGF levels in the mouse submandibular gland between E13 and postnatal day 21. Values are mean ± SEM and expressed as ng NGF/g wet weight. Data taken from Korsching and Thoenen (1988). The insert shows an enlargement of the early time points. Error bars smaller than symbol size were omitted. ●–● female and male organs pooled; ○–○ female gland; △–△ male gland.

(Thoenen and Barde, 1980). NGF in the superior cervical ganglion (SCG) (Fig. 5) was first detected at the same time as in its target organ, the submandibular gland. This is consistent with an almost immediate onset of retrograde axonal transport of NGF, once target contact is established. NGF content in the SCG then increased 21-fold during the next three days and continued to increase until the end of the third postnatal week, when adult levels were reached. Although the levels of NGF in the adult mouse submandibular gland are sexually dimorphic and 6 orders of magnitude higher than in other sympathetic target organs, no sex difference in the content was found either in the developing submandibular gland or the SCG until the end of the third postnatal week (Figs. 4 and 5). In addition, the steep NGF increase observed in the male submandibular gland after postnatal day 18 (250-fold within the following 3 days and up to 55000-fold in the next seven days) was not reflected in a corresponding increase in the NGF content of the male SCG. In accordance with earlier findings (Levi-Montalcini and Angeletti, 1968) it is concluded that neurons in the SCG do not have access to the large amounts of NGF synthesized during and after adolescence in the tubular duct cells of the mouse submandibular gland. It may be expected that the prepubertal NGF is synthesized in the acinar cells of the gland which are the ones receiving the sympathetic innervation.

These results support the concept that the initial fiber outgrowth and target contact of sympathetic neurons is not mediated by NGF. This is in accordance with the observation of Coughlin and Collins (1985) that sympathetic neurons begin to acquire dependance on NGF for survival only after E14, i.e. after the initial target contact. The function of NGF in early development then seems not to be the establishment of the correct innervation, but its stabilization and maintenance by regulating the survival of

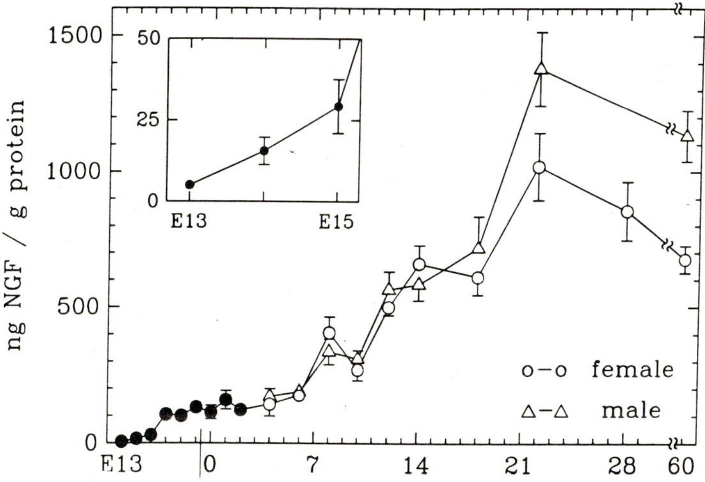

Figure 5. Developmental time course of NGF levels in the mouse SCG between E13 and 2 months of age. Values are mean ± SEM and expressed as ng NGF/g protein. Data taken from Korsching and Thoenen (1988). The insert shows an enlargement of the early time points. ●−● female and male organs pooled; ○−○ female SCG; △−△ male SCG.

30

these neurons. In addition, all results available so far are consistent with the concept that the fine-tuning of the innervation pattern, i.e. the innervation density of the different organs, could well be determined by their levels of NGF synthesis (Bjerre et al., 1975; Hopkins and Slack, 1984). The question remains: why do neurons have the ability of directed growth towards sources of NGF? Since chemotactic guidance by NGF is apparently not used in the establishment of innervation patterns, could NGF instead have a function in the repair of disturbed projections, i.e. during regeneration? As a first step to study this possibility we have examined the distribution of NGF and its mRNA after a lesion of the sciatic nerve, which contains both sensory and sympathetic axons besides the axons of motoneurons. Motoneurons, however, are not responsive to NGF (Thoenen and Barde, 1980).

The sciatic nerve of adult rats was cut at mid-thigh and the ends displaced to prevent regeneration. NGF and its mRNA levels were determined for up to 3 weeks after lesion, both distal and proximal to the cut, in five different segments spanning a total 2 cm. The NGF and mRNA^{NGF} content of the contralateral sciatic nerve was taken as the control, and it was not significantly different from that of untreated animals. The exceedingly high ratio of NGF to mRNA^{NGF} in the untreated sciatic nerve (300 vs about 10 for sympathetically innervated organs on a weight/weight basis, Heumann et al., 1987a) confirms the conclusion made earlier that most of the NGF found in the nerve is in transit, i.e. transported back by the axons, not synthesized locally in nonneuronal cells of the nerve. This is changed drastically by the cut. The mRNA for NGF shows a biphasic increase to maximally 14-fold over control values in the whole distal nerve stump and the proximal segment immediately adjacent to the cut. Some of the results are shown in Figure 6. The maximal increase was observed in the segment just distal to the cut, whereas NGF and its mRNA levels in the most proximal segment did not increase at all. The first increase of mRNA^{NGF} levels peaks already 6 h after cut; however, this increase seems not to result in the production of mature NGF. This is suggested by the observation that a cuff soaked with actinomycin D and cycloheximide blocks the increase in mRNA^{NGF}, but does not decrease the initial accumulation of NGF in section 3 (Heumann et al., 1987a). (The antibody used for determination of NGF most likely only recognizes the mature protein, cf. Barth et al., 1984). In addition, no increase in NGF protein is observed in the further distal segments 4 and 5 until 3 days after the cut, although the magnitude of the early increase in mRNA^{NGF} in these segments is quite comparable to that of the second phase. In fact the mechanism for the induction of mRNA^{NGF} seems to be different for the early and the late phase of mRNA^{NGF} induction. The initial increase, but not the later one, can be mimicked by placing a sciatic nerve explant in culture; however, addition of activated macrophages in culture can reproduce the second phase of mRNA^{NGF} induction (Heumann et al., 1987b). The second phase of mRNA^{NGF} increase reaches its maximum 3 days after cut for section 3 and even later for the more distal fragments. This rise in mRNA^{NGF} is accompanied by a corresponding rise in NGF protein in the segments 4 and 5 at a time when retrograde axonal transport of NGF has long ceased, i.e. 3 days after the cut. (In section 3 the experimental situation is less clear since we observe here an overlap of two independent phenomena, i.e. of NGF previously accumulated by retrograde transport and NGF that is locally synthesized at later time periods). It is concluded that in response to denervation the nonneuronal cells of the sciatic nerve begin to synthesize NGF. Moreover, the data for segment 2, directly proximal to the cut, suggest that the NGF synthesized locally is accessible to the cut axons. Here, mRNA^{NGF} is increased as much as in segment 3, however NGF itself does not increase above control values, suggesting that the NGF synthesized in this segment is removed by retrograde transport in the remaining axon stumps. When regeneration of the crushed sciatic nerve is allowed, the increase in NGF synthesis is reversible (Heumann et al., 1987b). These results raise the possibility that locally induced NGF synthesis could improve the regeneration of the severed sensory and sympathetic axons. Indeed, removal of endogenous NGF by injection of specific antibodies impaired considerably the regeneration of sympathetic neurons following lesion by 6-OH-

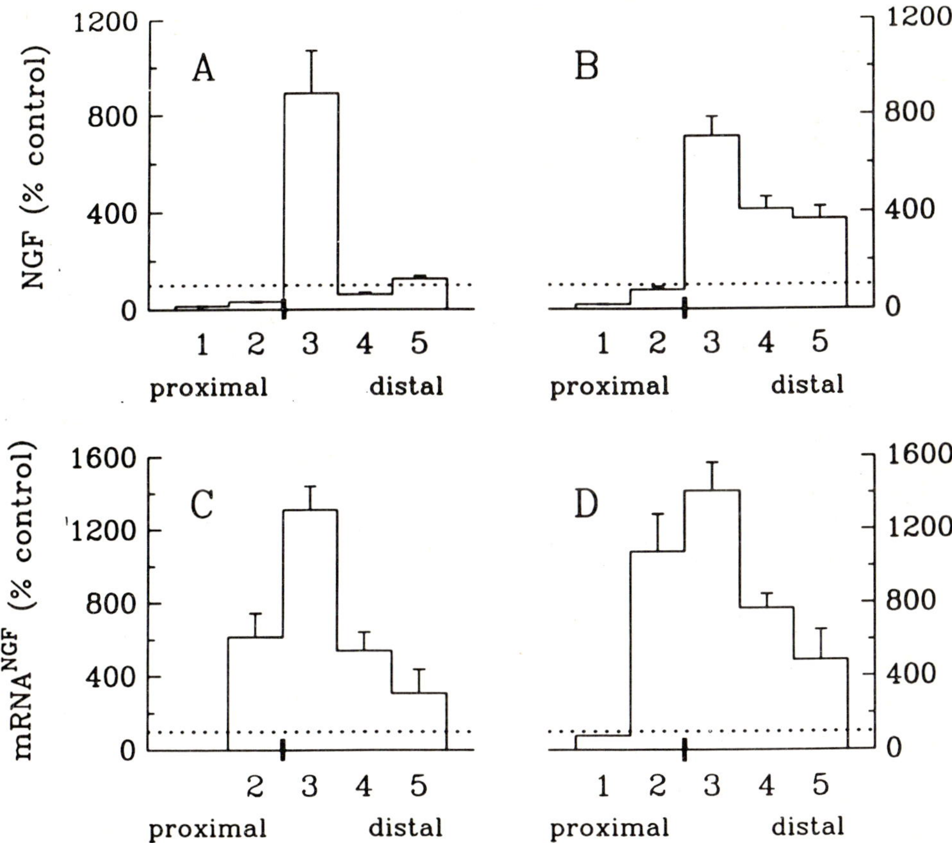

Figure 6. Long-term time course of NGF and mRNA^{NGF} levels in the sciatic nerve after a cut as indicated by the vertical bar between segment 2 and 3. The data are means ± SEM, taken from Heumann et al., 1987a, and expressed as % of contralateral control values. The stippled lines indicate the control value. A: NGF content 6h after cut (similar paradigm to Fig. 2B); B: NGF content 3 days after cut; C: mRNA^{NGF} 6h after cut; D: mRNA^{NGF} 3 days after cut.

dopamine (Bjerre et al., 1974). On the other hand, it has been observed that the regeneration of sensory axons is not influenced by autoimmunization against NGF (Rich et al., 1984). Further experiments will be needed to clarify this discrepancy.

It is interesting that NGF receptors are expressed in the denervated distal nerve stump with a time course similar to the induction of NGF synthesis (Taniuchi et al., 1986; Heumann et al., 1987b). These receptors are located on Schwann cells (see paper by Bandtlow et al., this volume). It is not yet clear, however, whether this might indicate an autocrine function of NGF for Schwann cells. An alternative possibility would be the restriction of diffusion of NGF by these, possibly low affinity-type, NGF receptors.

CONCLUSION

In conclusion, both NGF synthesis and expression of receptors for NGF are established at the time of initial target contact by sensory and sympathetic neurons. This seems to exclude the possibility that NGF could be used as chemotactic agent during initial target contact. However, NGF synthesis, induced locally in injured nerves, could serve to attenuate some effects of target organ deprivation.

REFERENCES

Barth E-M, Korsching S, Thoenen H (1984) Regulation of nerve growth factor synthesis and release in organ cultures of rat iris. J Cell Biol 99:839-843.

Bjerre B, Björklund A, Edwards DC (1974) Axonal regeneration of peripheral adrenergic neurons: effects of antiserum to nerve growth factor in mouse. Cell Tiss Res 148:441-476.

Bjerre B, Björklund A, Mobley W, Rosengren E (1975) Short- and long-term effects of nerve growth factor on the sympathetic nervous system in the adult mouse. Brain Res 94:263-277.

Coughlin MD, Collins MB (1985) Nerve growth factor-independent development of embryonic mouse sympathetic neurons in dissociated cell culture. Dev Biol 110:392-401.

Davies AM, Bandtlow C, Heumann R, Korsching S, Rohrer H, Thoenen H (1987) Timing and site of nerve growth factor synthesis in developing skin in relation to innervation and expression of the receptor. Nature 326:353-358.

Davies A, Lumsden A (1984) Relation of target encounter and neuronal death to nerve growth factor responsiveness in the developing mouse trigeminal ganglion. J Comp Neurol 223:124-137.

Gundersen RW, Barrett JN (1979) Neuronal chemotaxis: Chick dorsal root axons turn toward high concentrations of nerve growth factor. Science 206:1079-1080.

Heumann R, Korsching S, Bandtlow C, Thoenen H (1987a) Changes of nerve growth factor synthesis in nonneuronal cells in response to sciatic nerve transsection. J Cell Biol 104:1623-1631.

Heumann R, Lindholm D, Bandtlow C, Meyer M, Radeke MJ, Misko TP, Shooter EM, Thoenen H (1987b) Differential regulation of mRNA encoding nerve growth factor and its receptor in rat sciatic nerve during development, degeneration and regeneration: role of macrophages. Proc Natl Acad Sci USA 84: 8735-8739.

Heumann R, Korsching S, Scott J, Thoenen H (1984) Relationship between levels of nerve growth factor (NGF) and its messenger RNA in sympathetic ganglia and peripheral target tissues. EMBO J 3:3183-3189.

Heumann R, Thoenen H (1986) Comparison between the time course of changes in nerve growth factor protein levels and those of its messenger RNA in the cultured rat iris. J Biol Chem 261:9246-9249.

Holzbauer M, Sharman DF (1972) The distribution of catecholamines in vertebrates. Handbook of Experimental Pharmacology 33:110-185.

Hopkins WG, Slack JR (1984) Effect of nerve growth factor on intramuscular axons of neonatal mice. Neurosci 13:951-956.

Korsching S (1984) Thesis, Ludwig-Maximilians-Universität, München.

Korsching S (1986) Nerve growth factor in the central nervous system. Trends Neurosci 9:570-573.

Korsching S, Thoenen H (1983a) Nerve growth factor in sympathetic ganglia and corresponding target organs of the rat: Correlation with density of sympathetic innervation. Proc Natl Acad Sci USA 80:3513-3516.

Korsching S, Thoenen H (1983b) Quantitative demonstration of the retrograde axonal transport of endogenous nerve growth factor. Neurosci Lett 39:1-4.

Korsching S, Thoenen H (1985) Treatment with 6-OH-dopamine and colchicine decreases nerve growth factor levels in sympathetic ganglia and increases them in the corresponding target tissues. J Neurosci 5:1058-1061.

Korsching S, Thoenen H (1987) Two-site enzyme immunoassay for nerve growth factor. Meth Enzymol 147:167-185.

Korsching S, Thoenen H (1988) Developmental changes of nerve growth factor levels in sympathetic ganglia and their target organs. Dev Biol 126:40-46.

Levi-Montalcini R, Angeletti PU (1968) Nerve Growth Factor. Physiol Rev 48:534-569.

Levi-Montalcini R, Menesini Chen MG, Chen JS (1978) Neurotropic effects of the nerve growth factor in chick embryos and neonatal rodents. Zoon 6:201-212.

Palmatier MA, Hartmann BK, Johnson EM (1984) Demonstration of retrogradely transported endogenous nerve growth factor in axons of sympathetic neurons. J Neurosci 4:751-756.

Rich KM, Yip HK, Osborne PA, Schmidt RE, Johnson EM (1984) Role of nerve growth factor in the adult dorsal root ganglia neuron and its response to injury. J Comp Neurol 230:110-118.

Shelton DL, Reichardt LF (1984) Expression of the β-nerve growth factor gene correlates with the density of sympathetic innervation in effector organs. Proc Natl Acad Sci 81:7951-7955.

Shelton DL, Reichardt LF (1986) Studies on the regulation of β-nerve growth factor gene expression in the rat iris: The level of messenger RNA-encoding nerve growth factor is increased in irises placed in explant cultures *in vitro*, but not in irises deprived of sensory or sympathetic innervation *in vivo*. J Cell Biol 102:1940-1948.

Taniuchi M, Clark HB, Johnson EM (1986) Induction of nerve growth factor receptor in Schwann cells after axotomy. Proc Natl Acad Sci USA 83:4094-4098.

Thoenen H, Barde Y-A (1980) Physiology of nerve growth factor. Physiol Rev 60:1284-1335.

Neuronal Plasticity and Trophic Factors
G. Biggio, P.F. Spano, G. Toffano, S.H. Appel, G.L. Gessa (eds.)
Fidia Research Series, Symposia in Neuroscience VII
Liviana Press, Padova © 1988

CELLULAR LOCALIZATION OF NERVE GROWTH FACTOR SYNTHESIS IN VARIOUS ORGANS OF THE PERIPHERAL NERVOUS SYSTEM

C.E. Bandtlow, R. Heumann, M.E. Schwab and H. Thoenen

Max-Planck Institute for Psychiatry, Department of Neurochemistry,
Am Klopferspitz 18a, D-8033 Martinsried, F.R.G.
and Institute of Brain Research, August-Forelstr. 1,
CH-8029 Zürich, Switzerland

INTRODUCTION

The nerve growth factor (NGF) is as yet the only neurotrophic factor with an almost completely established physiological function, at least in the peripheral nervous system (Thoenen et al., 1987b).

NGF is essential for the development and maintenance of sympathetic and neural crest derived sensory neurons in the peripheral nervous system and, as recently shown, for magnocellular cholinergic neurons in the CNS (Thoenen et al, 1987a). However, the claim that NGF acted as a target derived neurotrophic factor was long based on the following indirect evidence:

— through a highly specific and saturable mechanism exogenous NGF is taken up by nerve terminals of responsive neurons and retrogradely transported to their pericarya (Hendry, 1980; Thoenen and Barde, 1980; Schwab et al., 1982);

— the administration of anti-NGF antibodies leads to the same effect as blockage of retrograde axonal transport (by chemical or mechanical methods), resulting in a destruction of sympathetic and sensory neurons in early periods of their development (Levi-Montalcini, 1968; Johnson, 1980; 1986) and impaired function in adult neurons

---

Abbreviations: NGF: Nerve growth factor, mRNA-NGF: messenger RNA of NGF, $[^{35}s]cRNA^{NGF+}$: anti sense strand transcript, $[^{35}s]cRNA^{NGF-}$: sense strand transcript.

(Gorin and Johnson, 1979; 1980; Rich et al., 1984), as reflected by a decrease in enzymes involved in the synthesis of Noradrenalin.

This indirect evidence has recently been further substantiated. In both the peripheral and central nervous systems there is a positive correlation between the levels of NGF and its mRNA on the one hand, and between these levels and the density of target field innervation by NGF responsive neurons on the other hand (Heumann et al., 1984; Korsching and Thoenen, 1983a; Shelton and Reichardt, 1986a). However, an important question about the biological function of NGF remained unanswered: what cell type or what cell types synthesize NGF in the various target organs. The answer could help us towards a better understanding of the mechanisms involved in the regulation of NGF synthesis. We chose to approach this question by using in situ hybridization, a technique originally developed by Gall and Pardue (1969) to detect rRNA. The method is in principle very similar to immunohistochemistry but, instead of radioactively labelled antibodies recombinant probes are used. However, even in the most densely innervated organs, NGF-mRNA is present at an extremely low copy number: less than one copy per million polyA$^+$-RNA molecules. Therefore not only is an optimal retention of cellular RNA-molecules required, but also probes with highly specific activities.

IN SITU HYBRIDIZATION

Methodology: Validation and Optimization of the Procedure

In previous experiments we used ^{32}-labelled, single stranded cRNA run-off transcripts (160-180 bases) or synthetic oligonucleotides (18-mer). However, the resolution of this isotope was unsatisfactory for a precise cellular localization. We therefore used ^{35}S-labelled probes, which have a much shorter path length but, unlike, tritiated probes, achieve a higher specific activity. Unexpectedly, we observed a marked unspecific binding of ^{35}S-labelled probes over sections as well as cultured cells. This unspecific binding was independent of the sequence and length of the probes (we used different cRNA probes and synthetic oligonucleotides). Even [^{35}S]αUTPs alone resulted in the same labelling pattern.

Moreover, neither an increase in the stringency of the washing conditions nor an extensive RNase treatment (100 μg/ml RNaseA and 10 μg/ml ribonuclease T1) after hybridization with cRNA probes reduced the unspecific binding. We therefore concluded that the substitution of an O with an S in the phosphate groups of the nucleotides led to a change in their chemical reactivity, probably resulting in a covalent binding to non-RNA-molecules. The specificity of the hybridization with ^{35}S-labelled probes was increased by:

— prehybridization of sections or cultured cells with non-labelled thioαUTPs;

— substitution of dithiothreitol (DTT) in the hybridization buffer by β-mercaptoethanol which is more stable to heat (hybridization at 50-55°C made an inactivation of the DTT likely);

— decreasing the pH of the hybridization buffer to pH5.5-6 (Fig. 1).

To prove that the specific signals were unaffected under the described conditions,

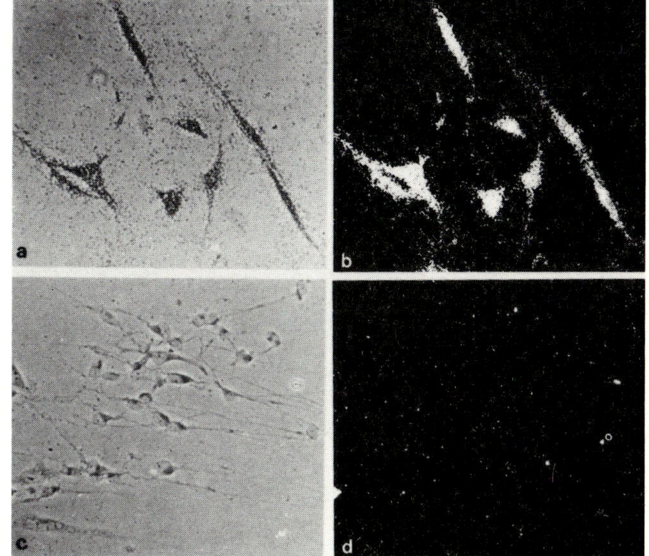

Figure 1. Phase contrast and corresponding darkfield photomicrographs showing unspecific binding of the [^{35}S] cRNA^{NGF-} (control) probe on sciatic nerve cells of newborn rats cultured for 24hrs, before (a+b) and after (c+d) pre-incubation with non-labelled thioαUTP (500nmoles/ml), β-mercaptoethanol at pH 5.5. Exposure time: 10 days.

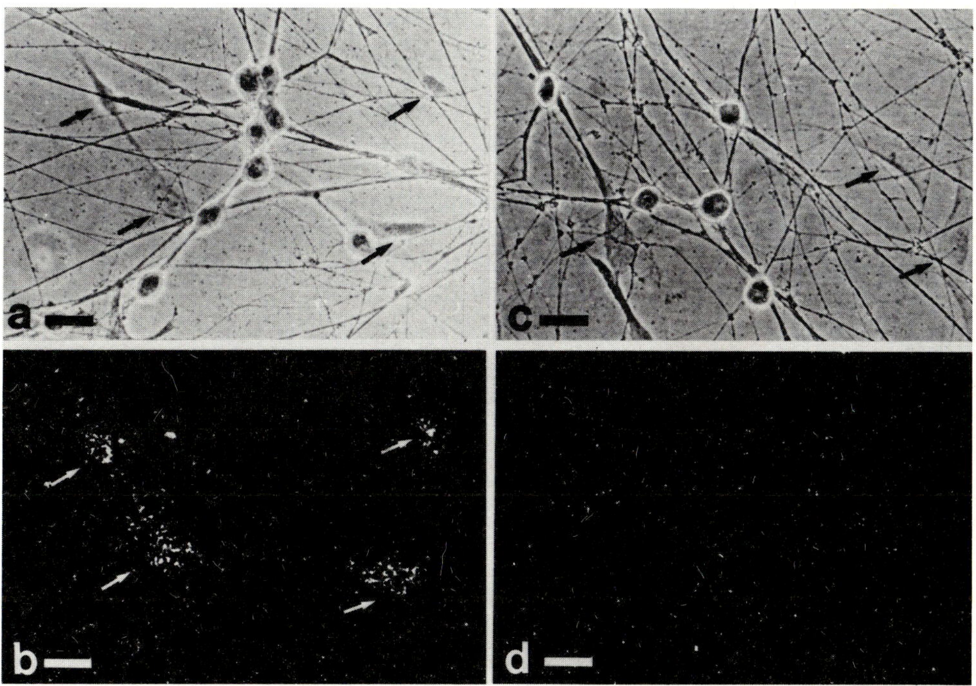

Figure 2. Phase contrast and darkfield photomicrographs of primary cultures of rat SCG. Only the non-neuronal cells are labelled (arrows) (a+b), whereas no specific labelling over cells is seen with the control probe (c+d). Exposure time: 18 days. Spacebar: 40 μm.

38

we used primary cultures from rat superior cervical ganglia, which besides sympathetic neurons, also consist of non-neuronal cells, like Schwann cells and fibroblasts. Hybridization of these cultures resulted in a specific labelling exclusively over non-neuronal cells, whereas the neurons were unlabelled (Fig. 2). These results not only showed that sympathetic neurons only respond to NGF but do not synthesize NGF-mRNA, they also support recent findings that the very high levels of NGF found in SCGs result from retrograde axonal transport (see Korsching, this volume).

Based on the biochemical data for NGF-mRNA levels in peripheral target organs (see Korsching, this volume) we chose the rat iris, the developing mouse whisker pad and the sciatic nerve as representative tissues for the cellular localization of NGF-mRNA with this improved in situ hybridization technique.

LOCALIZATION OF NGF-mRNA IN THE RAT IRIS

The native iris

The rat iris is an organ with a dense sympathetic, sensory and parasympathetic innervation (Hedlund et al., 1984). Investigations on the regional distribution of endogenous NGF indicated that the dilator region (mainly sympathetically innervated) has a 3-fold higher level of NGF than the sphincter region (predominantly cholinergic with relatively sparse adrenergic innervation) (Barth et al., 1984). A similar distribution was confirmed for NGF-mRNA levels (Shelton and Reichardt, 1986).

In agreement with these biochemical data, consistent labelling with $[^{35}S]cRNA^{NGF+}$ was observed over the ciliary body and along the posterior and anterior border layers on cryostat sections of native rat irides (Fig. 3). Ultrastructural studies (Hedlund et al., 1984) have demonstrated a very thin epithelial lining covering the posterior surface and a thicker, cuboidal epithelial cell layer covering the posterior side of the iris. The hybridization signals are mainly restricted to these areas, indicating that the epithelial cells do synthesize NGF-mRNA. However, the resolution of the method did not enable us to establish, whether, at the posterior side of the sections, the epithelial cell layer only was labelled or the underlying smooth muscle region as well. No signal above the background was seen over the mainly parasympathetically innervated sphincter region.

The cultured iris

Rat irides react upon culturing with an increase in the levels of endogenous NGF (Barth et al., 1984) reflected by a de novo synthesis of NGF-mRNA (Heumann et al., 1986; Shelton and Reichardt, 1986). These increased levels of NGF-mRNA were also observed in in situ hybridization experiments. A very intense signal was seen all over the sections, indicating that all major cell types produce NGF-mRNA (Fig. 3). Again the grain density was higher over the posterior layer, consisting of the cuboidal epithelial cell layer and the dilator region, than over the loose connective tissue at the anterior part. Moreover, the relative labelling intensity over the sphincter region was also lower, confirming recent data demonstrating that the relative NGF-mRNA content of the two muscle systems remained unchanged after culture (Shelton and Reichardt, 1986).

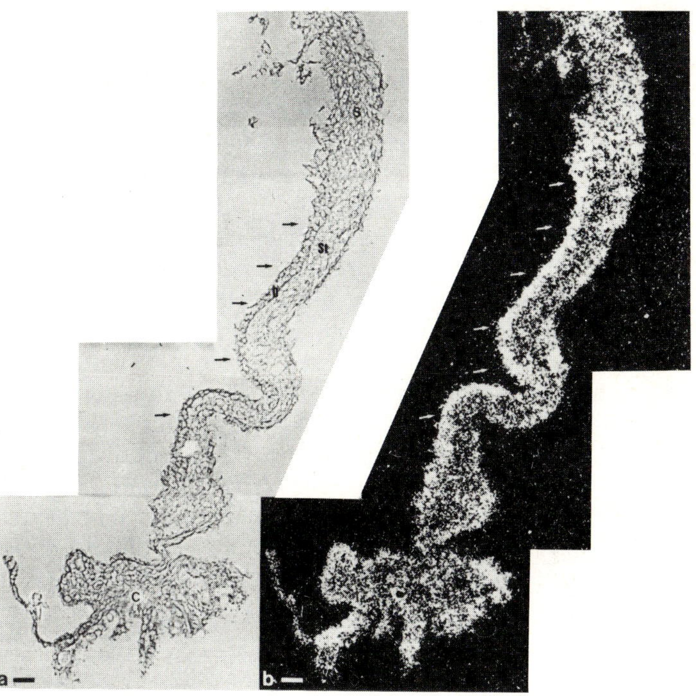

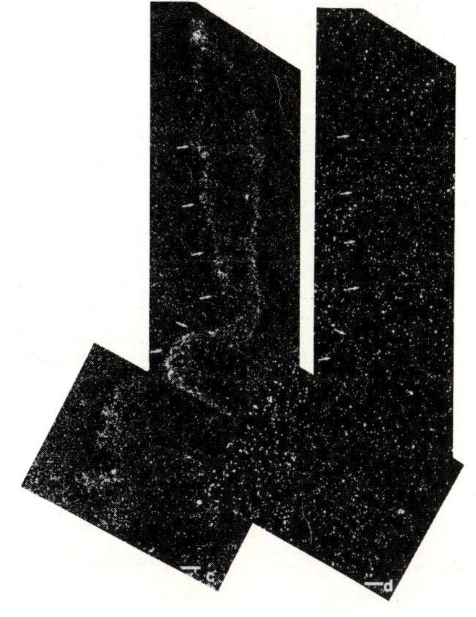

Figure 3. Localization of NGF-mRNA on cryostate sections of rat irides, hybridized with [^{35}S]cRNA^{NGF+}. (a) Phase contrast photomicrographs illustrating the smooth muscle regions: the mainly sympathetically innervated dilator (D), a one cell layer structure covered at the posterior part with a cuboidal epithelial cell layer (arrows), and the parasympathetically innervated sphincter (S). (C) ciliary body, (St) anterior stroma. (b) Darkfield photomicrographs of an induced iris (12 hrs in culture). Homogeneous distribution of grains over the anterior connective tissue, the sphincter and the ciliary body. The highest signal is found over the posterior border layer (arrows). (c) Darkfield photomicrographs of a native iris, with a specific signal restricted over the anterior and posterior border layers and parts of the ciliary body. (d) Darkfield photomicrographs illustrating the background grain density found over a cross section of a native iris, hybridized with [^{35}S]cRNA^{NGF-} (control).

Dissociated rat iris cell

Since our method did not allow a precise localization of the site of NGF synthesis, we studied the distribution of NGF-mRNA in primary cultures of rat irides. The cultures consist of smooth muscle cells, fibroblasts, epithelial cells and Schwann cells, as determined by specific immunocytochemical markers (Bandtlow et al., 1987). Virtually all cells were labelled, but with different signal intensities (Fig. 4). It was not possible to ascertain, whether the variations in signal intensity reflected a cell type specific difference of the NGF-mRNA content or resulted from variations in the accessability of NGF-mRNA sequences for the probes. However, these results indicate that NGF is not only synthesized by Schwann cells ensheathing NFG-responsive nerve fibers, as recently suggested by Rush (1986), but also — and to a much larger extent — by the target cells, i.e. epithelial cells, smooth muscle cells and fibroblasts. We have shown that binding of ^{125}J-NGF to dissociated rat iris cells occurs exclusively on Schwann cells, identified by a specific immunohistochemical marker (O_4) (Bandtlow et al., 1987). This observation led to the hypothesis that NGF produced by Schwann cells and other cell types could be bound by the Schwann cell receptors (and even accumulated by internalization) thereby resulting in detectable staining with anti-NGF antibodies of Schwann cells only.

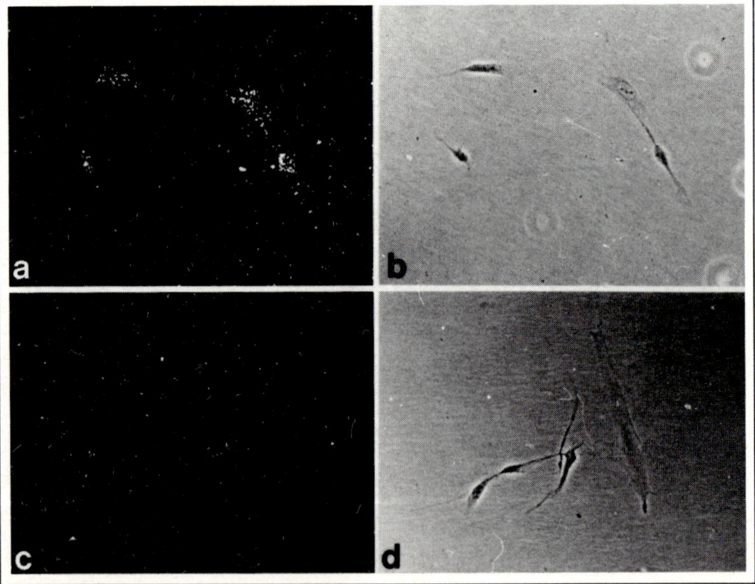

Figure 4. Primary culture of adult rat irides, 24 hrs in culture (a + b). Phase contrast and darkfield photomicrographs showing specific signals with different intensities over all cells hybridized with [^{35}S]cRNA^{NGF+}; no signal above background is seen after hybridization with [^{35}S]cRNA^{NGF-} (control). Exposure time was 16 days. Spacebar: 40 μm.

LOCALIZATION OF NGF-mRNA
IN THE DEVELOPING MOUSE WHISKER PAD

The mouse whisker pad was used as an example of an exclusively sensory innervated target organ. Recent findings suggest that initial target-field innervation is correlated with the onset of NGF-mRNA synthesis (Davies et al. 1987; see also Korsching, this volume). We therefore considered two different developmental stages: at E10, before the fibers have reached their target, and at E13 where emerging fibers from the trigeminal ganglion reach their maximal target-field contact (Davies et al., 1987; see also Korsching, this volume).

In line with the biochemical data, hybridization of sections at E10 gave no detectable signals over the maxillary process (Fig. 5). However, in agreement with the finding that the concentration of NGF and its mRNA at E13 is higher in the epithelium than in the mesenchyme (Davies et al, 1987), hybridizing sections of the E13 mouse whisker pad with $[^{35}S]cRNA^{NGF+}$ showed a higher labelling of the epithelium than of the central mesenchyme. The silver grain density was equally distributed over both the surface and the follicular epithelium along with their adjacent mesenchyme (Fig. 6). Since the resolution of the in situ hybridization did not allow us to unequivocally identify individual cells, it was not possible to ascertain whether all epithelial cells synthesize

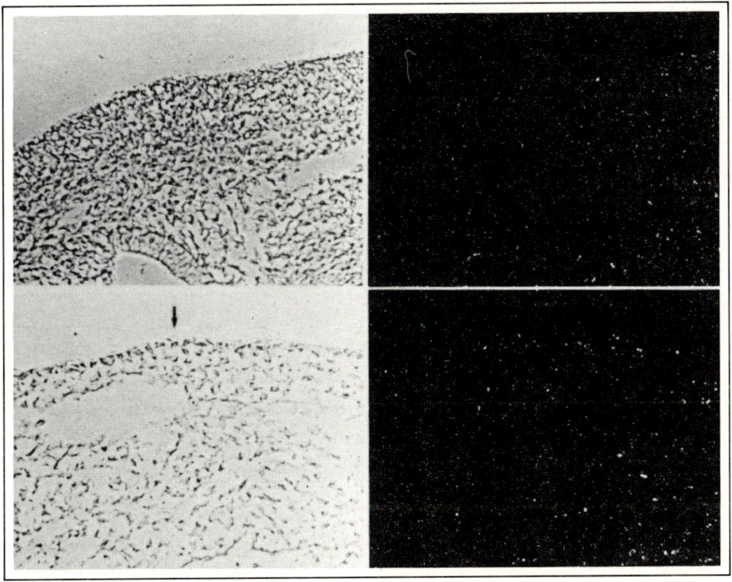

Figure 5. Localization of NGF-mRNA over paraffin sections through a mouse head at E10. (a + b) phase contrast and darkfield photomicrographs of a section showing no specific signal above background over the maxillary process (arrow). (c + d) corresponding control section (b). Exposure time was 20 days. Spacebar: 100 µm.

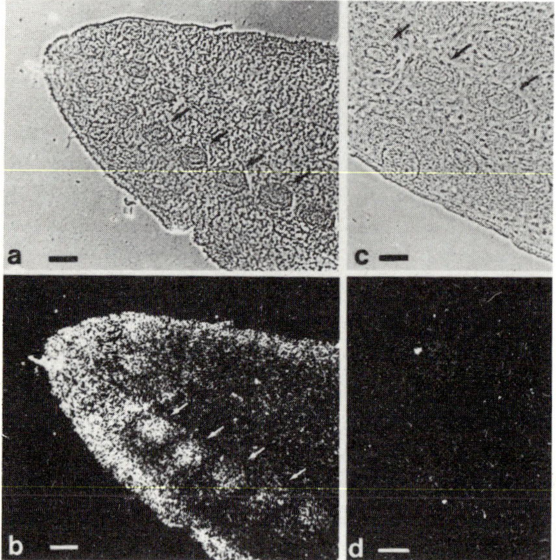

Figure 6. Localization of NGF-mRNA over paraffin sections through a mouse whisker pad at E13. (a + b) phase contrast and darkfield photomicrographs of a section passing a row of whisker follicles (arrows); both the follicular and surface epithelium with their adjacent mesenchyme are densely labelled, whereas the central mesenchyme shows more moderate labelling throughout. (c + d) corresponding control sections. Exposure time was 20 days. Spacebar: 100 µm.

NGF-mRNA. Nonetheless, there was no obvious regional distribution pattern within the epithelium; both the surface and follicular epithelium were heavily labelled. Although the mesenchyme of the whisker pad was labelled throughout, the region just beneath the surface epithelium was more heavily labelled. Since this region gives rise to the dermis, the distribution of NFG-mRNA in the mesenchyme reflects the termination of nerve fibers, which are more numerous in the dermis than in subcutaneous tissues. This observation further supports the concept that NGF synthesis occurs predominantly in the target tissues of NGF-responsive neurons and certainly does not depend exclusively upon the Schwann cells ensheathing them.

LOCALIZATION OF NGF-mRNA IN ADULT RAT SCIATIC NERVES AFTER TRANSECTION

The transection of the sciatic nerve leads to marked changes in the levels of NGF and in its mRNA, both distal and proximal to the transection site (Heumann et al., 1987; see also Korsching, this volume). In situ hybridization experiments have demonstrated that NGF-mRNA distal to the transection site is homogenously distributed over longitudinal sections prepared 4d after cutting (Fig. 7). This homogeneous labelling (the epineurium was generally weakly labelled) indicates that not only the non-neuronal cells surrounding the axons of sympathetic and sensory neurons but also those ensheathing motor neurons, contain NGF-mRNA.

The events taking place proximal to the transection site are of particular interest with respect to the initiation of the regeneration of NGF responsive nerve fibers. Unlike

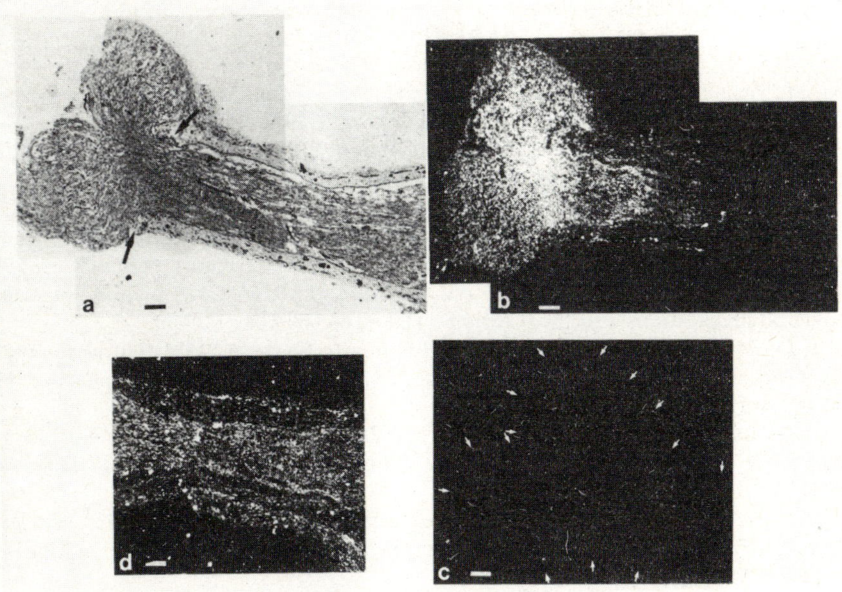

Figure 7. Localization of NGF-mRNA over cryostate longitudinal sections of adult rat sciatic nerves 4d after transection. Phase contrast (a) and darkfield photomicrographs (b) of a section through the proximal nerve stump, showing dense labelling over the neuroma-like structure (arrows) and over the adjacent 2.4 mm of the proximal part of the stump. No detectable signal is seen over the residual proximal part of the nerve stump. (c) longitudinal section through the distal part of the transected nerve shows a homogeneous grain distribution throughout the section. (d) corresponding control section of the proximal stump; arrows indicate che neuroma-like structure. Exposure time was 22 days: Spacebar: 0.4 mm.

the extensive NGF-mRNA changes in the distal nerve stump, the changes in the proximal nerve part are strictly confined to the immediately adjacent nerve part of the transection site (Heumann et al., 1987). Moreover, in situ hybridization showed that 4 days after cutting the most intense labelling was seen in a neuroma-like structure, containing outgrowing neurites and co-migrating cells (Fig. 7). It is reasonable to consider this end of the proximal nerve stump a "substitute target", where NGF synthesized by non-neuronal cells is available to support the regeneration of NGF-responsive fibers.

ACKNOWLEDGMENTS

We are grateful to Cheryl Mc Caffrey for her critical reading of the manuscript. The research project was supported in part by the Deutsche Forschungsgemeinschaft.

REFERENCES

Bandtlow CE, Heumann R, Schwab ME, Thoenen H (1987) Cellular localization of nerve growth factor synthesis by in situ hybridization. EMBO J 6: 891-899.

Barth E-M, Korsching S, Thoenen H (1984) Regulation of nerve growth factor synthesis and release in organ cultures of rat iris. J Cell Biol 99:839-843.

Davies AM, Bandtlow CE, Heumann R, Korsching S, Rohrer H, Thoenen H (1987a) The site and timing of nerve growth factor (NGF) synthesis in developing skin in relation to its innervation by sensory neurons and their expression of NGF receptors. Nature 326: 353-363.

Gall JG, Pardue MC (1969) Formation and detection of RNA-DNA hybrid molecules in cytological preparations. Proc Natl Acad Sci (USA) 64:600-604.

Hedlund K-O, Ayer-Lelievre C, Björklund H, Hultgren L, Seiger A (1984) Ultrastructural and histochemical studies of the rat iris: identified neuronal inputs and supportive glia. J Neurocytol 13:703-725.

Heumann R, Korsching S, Scott J, Thoenen H (1984) Relationship between levels of nerve growth factor (NGF) and its messenger RNA in sympathetic ganglia and peripheral target tissues. EMBO J 3:3183-3189.

Heumann R, Thoenen H (1986) Comparison between time course of changes in nerve growth factor (NGF) protein levels and those of its messenger RNA in the cultured iris. J Biol Chem 261:9246-9249.

Heumann R, Korsching S, Bandtlow C, Thoenen H (1987a) Changes of nerve growth factor synthesis in non-neuronal cells in response to sciatic nerve transection. J Cell Biol 104:1623-1631.

Korsching S, Thoenen H (1983a) Nerve growth factor in sympathetic ganglia and corresponding target organs of the rat: correlation with density of sympathetic innervation. Proc Natl Acad Sci (USA) 80:3513-3516.

Rush RH (1984) Immunohistochemical localization of endogenous nerve growth factor. Nature 312:364-367.

Shelton D, Reichardt L (1984) Expression of nerve growth factor gene correlates with the density of sympathetic innervation in effector organs. Proc Natl Acad Sci (USA) 81:7951-7955.

Shelton D, Reichardt L (1986b) Studies on the regulation of beta-nerve growth factor gene expression in the rat iris: The level of mRNA-encoding nerve growth factor is increased in irises placed in explant cultures in vitro, but not in irises deprived of sensory or sympathetic innervation in vivo. J Cell Biol 102:1940-1948.

Thoenen H, Auburger G, Hellweg R, Heumann R, Korsching S (1987a) Cholinergic innervation and levels of nerve growth factor and its mRNA in the central nervous system. In: Cholinergic Mechanisms, Vol. 6. Cellular and Molecular Basis of Cholinergic Function. Ellis Horwood, Chichester, in press.

Neuronal Plasticity and Trophic Factors
G. Biggio, P.F. Spano, G. Toffano, S.H. Appel, G.L. Gessa (eds.)
Fidia Research Series, Symposia in Neuroscience VII
Liviana Press, Padova © 1988

STUDIES ON A GENE SEQUENCE WHOSE EXPRESSION IS REGULATED BY NGF IN PC12 CELLS

A. Levi, R. Possenti, J. Eldridge[1] and B.M. Paterson[1]

Institute of Neurobiology, CNR, Via Romagnosi 18a, 00196 Roma, Italy,
and [1]Laboratory of Biochemistry, National Cancer Institute,
National Institutes of Health, Bethesda, MD 20892, USA

INTRODUCTION

The protein NGF is an essential trophic and differentiative factor for peripheral sympathetic and sensory neurones of vertebrates (Levi Montalcini, 1966; Cohen et al., 1954) and for a subpopulation of neurones in the central nervous system (Korsching et al., 1985; Mobley et al., 1985). Moreover, other cell types, derived from the neural crest, respond to NGF. Adrenal medullary cells, for instance, acquire a neuronal phenotype, in vivo and in vitro, when exposed to the factor (Aloe and Levi Montalcini, 1979; Unsicker et al., 1978). PC12 cells, a line derived from a rat phaeochromocytoma, have maintained the property of their untransformed counterpart of differentiating in the presence of NGF, assuming several properties of a mature sympathetic neurone (Greene and Tischler, 1976). Since PC12 are a clonal population of cells that can be harvested in large quantities, they have been the most convenient system for biochemical studies on the mechanism of action of NGF. The process of NGF-induced differentiation of PC12 cells requires de novo synthesis of RNA and most likely expression of new gene products (Burstein and Greene, 1978). In fact, several reports describe early and delayed changes in the level of distinct proteins in PC12 cells exposed to NGF (McGuire and Greene, 1980; Dickson et al., 1986; Tiercy and Shooter, 1986).

In order to further investigate the role of NGF-induced modulation of gene expression in PC12 cells we decided to obtain cDNA probes for NGF-inducible genes. To this aim, we generated a cDNA library from mRNA of PC12 cells treated for 24 hours with NGF. We have previously described the isolation from such a cDNA library of a clone named VGF hybridizing to a mRNA induced approximately 50 fold by NGF with a dose dependence that parallels the NGF binding to its receptors (Levi et al., 1985). Here we present extended studies as well as new data on the characterization of the VGF RNA, the modulation of its expression in PC12 cells and in other cell lines and we show preliminary data on the structure and localization of the protein coded by the VGF gene.

RESULTS

Northern blot analysis of RNA derived from PC12 cells after different periods of treatment with NGF shows that the level of VGF mRNA increases considerably (Fig. 1 A, B). Quantitative determinations on this and similar experiments may be summarized as follows:

— the induction of VGF mRNA due to NGF is a relatively early event as its level is already well above the control after three hours;

— it reaches a maximum (fifty to eighty fold increase) between six to nine hours; and

— VGF mRNA is present in high amount, comparable to the one of actin, also in cells that are fully differentiated.

Different molecular mechanisms may account for the accumulation of VGF mRNA induced by NGF: in particular, it may be due to higher transcription rate or higher RNA stability or both. A way to distinguish, at least in part, between these possibilities is offered by run-on experiments. According to this procedure, nuclei are isolated from the cells, the total nascent RNA is labelled in vitro and a specific sequence is evidentiated by its hybridization to a complementary DNA immobilized on nitrocellulose paper. The strength of the hybridization signal is a measure of the rate of synthesis of the specific RNA. Figure 2 shows that there is about ten fold more RNA complementary to VGF cDNA synthesized on nuclei isolated from PC12 treated for 6 hours with NGF than on nuclei isolated from untreated cells. This means that at least part of the effect of NGF on the induction of VGF is due to transcriptional control. Consequently we decided to look, at the level of the genome, for DNA sequences responsible for the inducibility of VGF by NGF. Using VGF cDNA as a probe we screened a rat genomic library in lamda Charon 4a and isolated from a number of phages representing approximately five genomes three independent phages sharing common sequences according to restriction analysis. From one of these phages we subcloned a five Kbp long Hind III restriction fragment (named Hg) that contained all the information present in VGF cDNA. Sequences homologous to the TATA and CAAT consensus sequences are present in the genomic clone respectively 30 bp and 70 bp 5' to the start of transcription. Detailed information on the genomic sequence of VGF will be presented elsewhere.

A schematic representation of the gene is presented in Figure 3 together with the constructs of hybrid genes coding for the chloroamphenicol acetyl transferase gene (CAT) under control of the VGF promoter used in expression studies after transfection. These two hybrid genes were used to investigate two main aspects of the VGF gene regulation, i.e. the induction of its transcription by NGF and the cell specificity of its

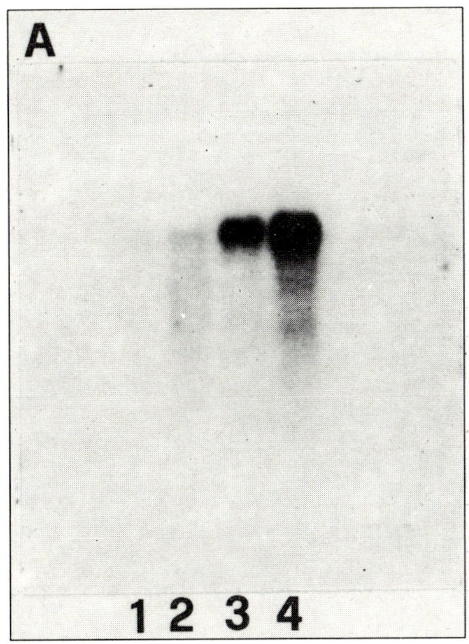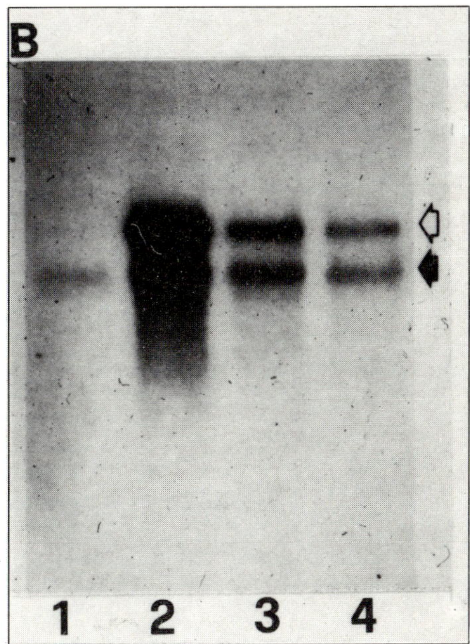

Figure 1. Northern analysis of RNA from NGF treated and control PC12 cells. 10 µg of RNA isolated from PC12 cells exposed to 100 ng/ml of NGF was subjected to electrophoresis in denaturing conditions, blotted and hybridized to nick translated probes. A: RNA extracted from cells treated with NGF for 0, 1, 3 and 6 hours (lanes 1, 2, 3, 4 respectively) hybridized with nick translated VGF probe. B: RNA extracted from cells treated with NGF for 0, 2, 10 and 14 days (lanes 1, 2, 3 and 4 respectively). The open arrow points to the hybridization signal due to the VGF probe, the black arrow points to the signal due to a rat actin probe used as an internal reference.

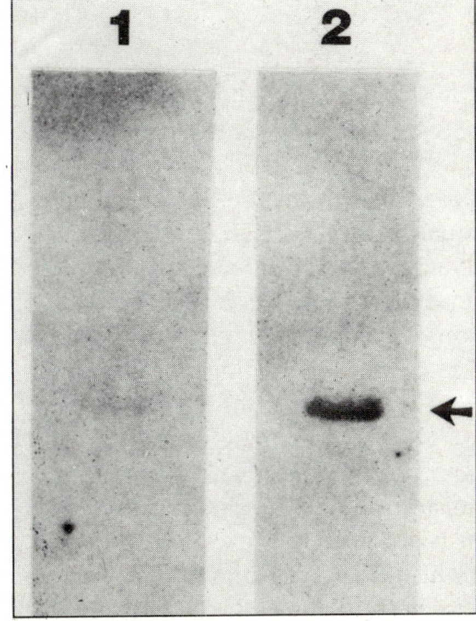

Figure 2. Transcription of VGF RNA from nuclei isolated from control and NGF treated cells. Nuclei were isolated from control PC12 cells (1) and cells treated with 100 ng/ml of NGF for 6 hours (2). Nascent RNA was labelled in the presence of P32 UTP. Equal amounts of counts from the reactions were hybridized to VGF e cDNA immobilized on nitrocellulose paper (marked by the arrow).

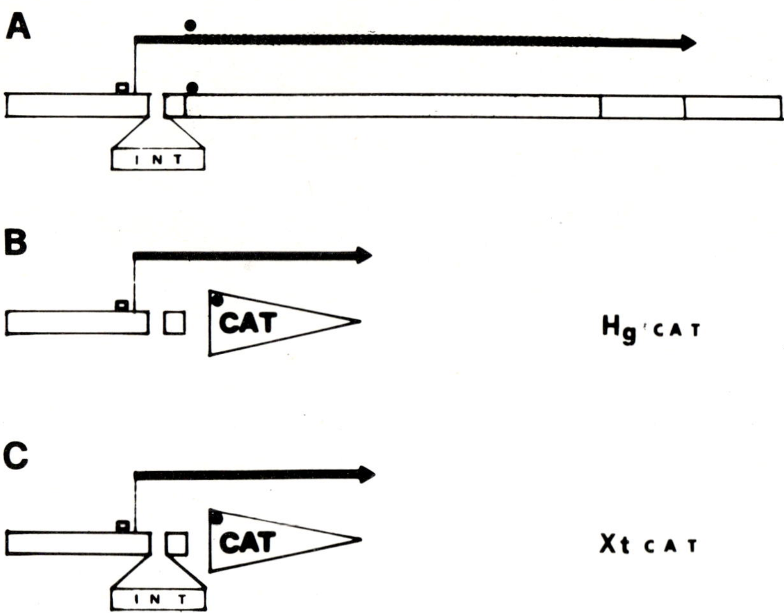

Figure 3. Diagram of the VGF gene and the constructs used in transfection experiments. A represents the genomic fragment coding for the VGF mRNA; B and C show the two constructs used to measure the promoter activity of the VGF gene in transfection experiments. The intron in the non coding leader sequence (int in A and C) has been deleted in Hg-CAT (B). The open squares indicate the TATA consensus sequence, the black arrows depict the mRNA, and the open circles indicate the beginning of the protein coding region.

expression. The first construct named Hg-CAT was obtained by splicing in front of the bacterial CAT gene a fragment of Hg starting about 0.7 kb 5' to the start of the VGF RNA and terminating about 50 bp inside the VGF RNA. The second construct (Xt-CAT) was made to determine whether the single intron present in the leader sequence of the VGF gene plays a role in the control of its expression. We took advantage of a XmnI site present in the VGF sequence 5 bp after the first in frame AUG and by trimming these 5 bp we were able to obtain a fusion gene having not only the promoter region of Hg but also the whole leader sequence of the VGF RNA spliced in front of the CAT coding region.

A typical result of CAT assay after transient transfection of Hg-CAT and Xt-CAT in PC12 is presented in Figure 4. Due to the non specific general activation of transcription and translation induced by NGF in PC12 cells the activity due to transfection of a plasmid in which the CAT gene is under control of the Rous Sarcoma Virus promoter was used as a reference. Figure 5 shows the result of a similar experiment in which RSV-CAT and Xt-CAT were transfected in different cell lines namely PC12, C2 (a rat derived miogenic cell line) and L cells (a mouse fibroblast cell line).

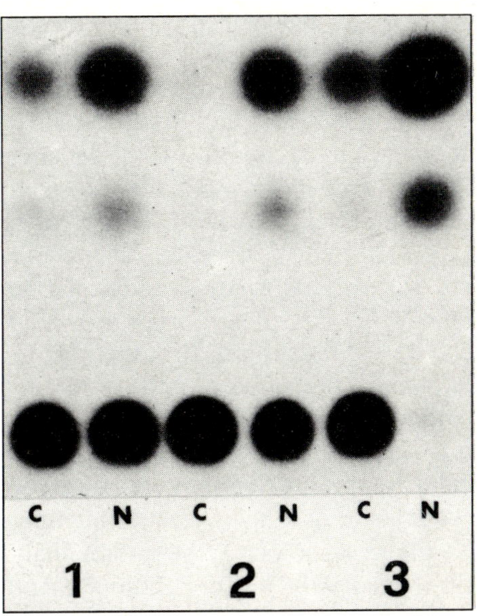

Figure 4. Hg-CAT and Xt-CAT expression in transfected PC12 cells. PC12 cells were transiently transfected with CAT constructs containing the RSV promoter (lanes 1) or the putative promoter region of the VGF gene without (Hg-CAT lanes 2) or with (Xt-CAT lanes 3) the single VGF intron. Cells were exposed to 100 ng/ml of NGF 24 hours before the preparation of the extracts. C and N represent extracts from control and NGF treated cells respectively. In lanes 1 ten times less extract than in 2 and 3 was used.

The result of these studies may be summarized as follows:

— the difference between Hg-CAT and Xt-CAT in terms of CAT activity after transfection in PC12 cells is only quantitative and not qualitative since both Hg-CAT and Xt-CAT are up regulated in their expression by the NGF even after compensating for the overall pleitrophic effect of this factor. The amount of induction by NGF is, however, much less than in the case of the endogenous gene;

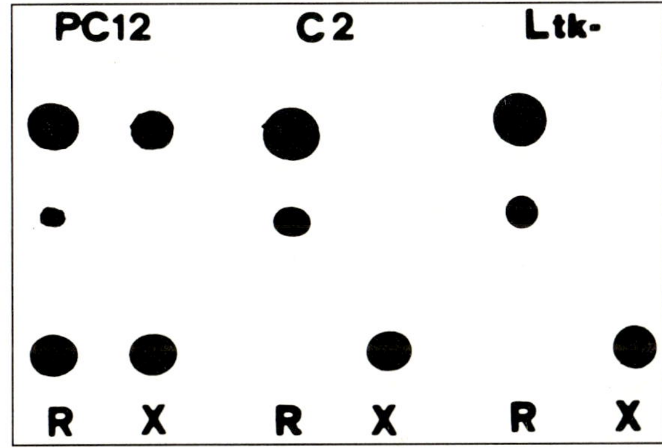

Figure 5. Expression of transfected Xt-CAT in different cell lines. PC12 cells, C2 cells and L cells were transiently transfected with RSV-CAT (lanes R) or Xt-CAT (lanes X) and assayed for CAT activity after two days. For each cell line the same amount of protein was used in the assay.

50

— PC12 cells which express the endogenous VGF gene express the hybrid CAT construct better than other cell lines. Several explanations, currently under experimental investigation, may account for the modest level of activation of Hg-CAT and Xt-CAT by NGF in PC12 cells. A first possibility is that DNA regions acting as NGF-inducible enhancers are located outside the genomic fragments used in the CAT hybrid constructs. It is also conceivable that the transiently transfected DNA is not able to mimic the endogenous gene because it is in a different conformation not being integrated in the genome. Moreover, since several copies of the transfected gene are taken up by the cells they may saturate whatever molecular mechanism is mediating intracellularly the effect of the NGF.

In a different set of experiments we sought to acquire information on the biochemical properties and the intracellular localization of the VGF gene product with the aim of understanding its function. Antisera directed against the VGF antigen were obtained in rabbits by injecting fusion proteins expressed in E. Coli. These proteins were made by splicing different portions of the VGF cDNA in front of the bacterial beta-galactosidase in a plasmid containing an inducible promoter.

Figure 6 shows a Western blot analysis of cell extracts from control PC12 cells and cells treated with NGF for 24 hours. Antisera directed against a different portion of the VGF protein gave the same pattern of staining as well as sera preadsorbed on the beta galactosidase. On the contrary the reactivity with PC12 extract could be abolished by preadsorbing the sera against recombinant VGF protein expressed in bacteria (data not shown). Two major bands with a molecular weight of about 80,000 Dalton are evidentiated by the antibodies. We tend to believe that this doublet arises by post-translational modification in vivo since it is present even when the cells are lysed in conditions that should minimize proteolysis.

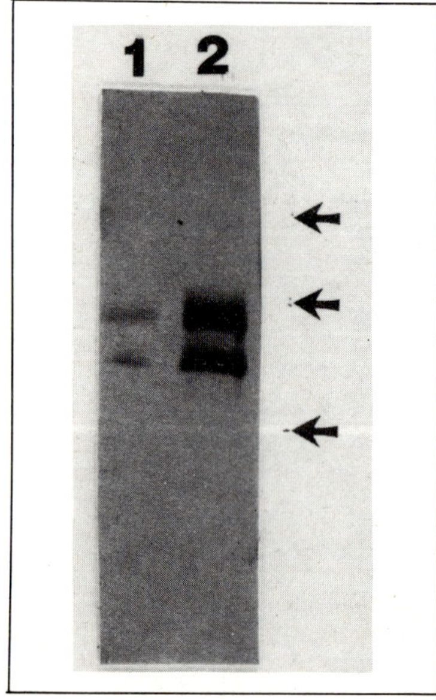

Figure 6. Western blot analysis of PC12 proteins probed with antibodies against VGF. Extracts from PC12 cells were electrophoresed on 7.5% SDS polyacrylamide gel. Proteins were transferred to nitrocellulose membranes and analyzed with antisera against VGF protein. Lane 1: extracts from control PC12 cells. Lane 2: extracts from cells treated with 100 ng/ml of NGF for 24 hours. The arrows indicate the position of molecular weight markers: from top to bottom 116.25, 97.4, 66.2 K Dalton.

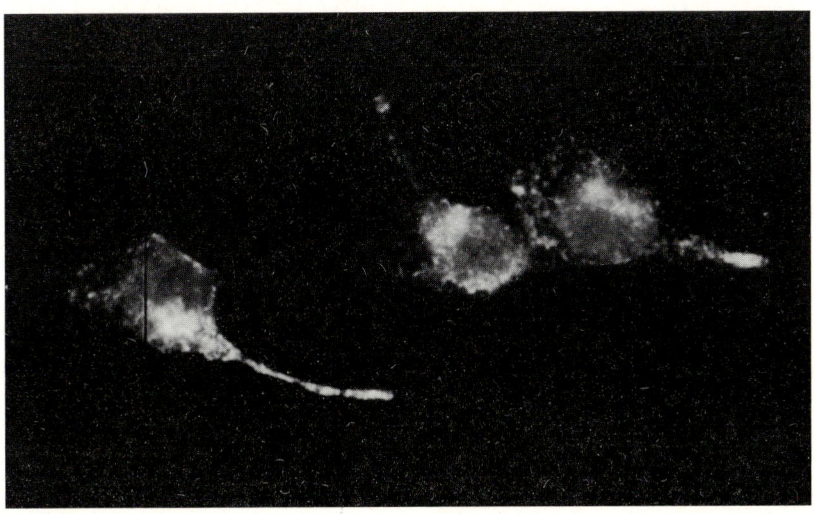

Figure 7. Indirect immunofluorescent staining of PC12 cell with antibodies directed against VGF protein. PC12 cells grown for 48 hours in the presence of 100 ng/ml of NGF were fixed, permeabilized and treated with rabbit antisera directed against VGF protein. Antibodies binding was visualized by staining with fluorescein-conjugated goat anti-rabbit antibodies.

Preliminary experiments aimed at determinating the intracellular localization of the VGF by immunofluorescence are shown in Figure 7. The staining is evident only in permeabilized cells and is compatible with the VGF antigen being associated with subcellular organells. This finding is substantiated by cell fractionation experiments that indicate that the VGF antigen is sedimentable at $100,000 \times g$ (data not shown).

CONCLUSIONS

PC12 cells are an interesting model for the study of neuronal differentiation since they respond to a factor (the NGF) that is essential for the differentiation of precursor cells to mature neurones in vivo. If we define the process of cell differentiation as the coordinate expression (or repression) of specific sets of genes, it is clear the utility of acquiring molecular probes for such genes.

In this paper we have described some of the properties of a gene named VGF coding for a mRNA that is induced several fold in PC12 cells by NGF. Increased level of VGF is an early response of PC12 cells to NGF and is at least partially accounted for by an induction of transcription. Some of the DNA sequences responsible for conferring NGF-inducibility to the VGF gene in PC12 cells are located within 0.7 kb 5' to the start of the RNA. The same region spliced in front of an indicator gene allows its expression in PC12 cell to a much higher level than in other "non neuronal" cell lines. We tentatively assume that this 0.7 Kbp region is target for positive regulation by factors present in PC12 cells and modulated by NGF. It is clear, however, that this sequence is not sufficient per se in conferring to a transfected gene the same NGF-inducibility as the endogenous gene. Understanding which ones are the molecular events responsible for this discrepancy will hopefully help to shed light on the mode of action of NGF.

A different kind of tool is provided by the antibodies against the VGF antigen. They will help to understand whether the VGF protein plays a causative role in the subsequent events leading to the PC12 differentiation or whether it simply represents a marker of the neuronal phenotype shared by differentiated PC12 and, as preliminary data show, by subsets of neurones in the central nervous system.

ACKNOWLEDGMENTS

We are grateful to Dr. Don Court for providing the vectors used for expressing recombinant VGF protein in E. Coli. This work was partially supported by research grant Progetto Strategico Neurobiologia Cellulare e Molecolare.

REFERENCES

Aloe L, Levi Montalcini R (1979) Nerve growth factor-induced transformation of immature chromaffin cells into sympathetic neurons: effects of antiserum to nerve growth factor. Proc Natl Acad Sci USA 76:1246-1250.

Burstein DE, Greene LA (1978) Evidence for RNA synthesis-dependent and -independent pathways in stimulation of neurite outgrowth by nerve growth factor. Proc Natl Acad Sci USA 75:6059-6053.

Cohen S, Levi Montalcini R, Hamburger V (1954) A nerve growth-stimulating factor isolated from sarcoma 37 and 180. Proc Natl Acad Sci USA 40:1014-1018.

Dickson G, Prentice H, Julien JP, Ferrari G, Leon A, Walsh FS (1986) Nerve growth factor activates thy-1 and neurofilament gene transcription in rat PC12 cells. EMBO Journal 5:3449-3453.

Greene LA, Tishler AS (1976) Establishment of a noradrenergic clonal line of rat adrenal, pheochromocytoma cells which respond to nerve growth factor. Proc Natl Acad Sci USA 73:2424-2428.

Korshing S, Auberger G, Heumann R, Scott J, Thoenen H (1985) Levels of nerve growth factor and its mRNA in the central nervous system of rat correlate with cholinergic innervation. EMBO Journal 4:1389-1393.

Levi A, Eldridge JD, Paterson BM (1985) Molecular cloning of a gene sequence regulated by nerve growth factor. Science 229:393-395.

Levi Montalcini R (1966) The nerve growth factor: its mode of action on sensory and sympathetic nerve cells. Harvey Lecture 60:217-248.

McGuire JC, Greene LA (1980) Stimulation by nerve growth factor of specific protein synthesis in rat PC12 pheochromocytoma cells. Neuroscience 5:179-189.

Mobley WC, Rutkowsky JL, Tennekoon GI, Buchanan K, Johnston MV (1985) Choline acetyltransferase activity in striatum of neonatal rats increased by nerve growth factor. Science 229:284-287.

Tiercy JM, Shooter EM (1986) Early changes in the synthesis of nuclear and cytoplasmic proteins are induced by nerve growth factor in differentiating rat PC12 cells. The Journal of Cell Biology 103:2367-2378.

Unsicker K, Kirsch B, Otten U, Thoenen H (1978) Nerve growth factor-induced fiber outgrowth from isolated rat adrenal chromaffin cells: impairment by glucocorticoids. Proc Natl Acad Sci USA 75:3498-3502.

Neuronal Plasticity and Trophic Factors
G. Biggio, P.F. Spano, G. Toffano, S.H. Appel, G.L. Gessa (eds.)
Fidia Research Series, Symposia in Neuroscience VII
Liviana Press, Padova © 1988

THE CONTROL OF CELL GROWTH AND DIFFERENTIATION BY FIBROBLAST GROWTH FACTOR

Denis Gospodarowicz and Napoleone Ferrara

Cancer Research Institute, University of California Medical Center,
San Francisco, California, USA

INTRODUCTION

Over the last 4 years, both basic and acidic fibroblast growth factors (bFGF and aFGF) have been purified to homogeneity, their primary structures determined, and their cDNA cloned and sequenced (Gospodarowicz et al., 1986a; 1986b; Baird et al., 1986; Abraham et al., 1987). This information has had significant impact on our understanding of a variety of mitogenic activities isolated from diverse origin. It has become clear that growth factors isolated from ovary, adrenal, kidney, eye, brain, placenta, macrophages, prostate, cartilage, and various tumors, are structurally and biologically identical, or at least, very similar to bFGF or aFGF (Gospodarowicz et al., 1986a). Availability of the pure mitogens has led to the recognition of a wide spectrum of activities for these two factors (Gospodarowicz, 1985), most notably, their ability to mimic the biological effect of the vegetalizing factor in early embryos (Slack et al., 1987) and to act as angiogenic factors. Basic FGF or aFGF are multifunctional, since they can both stimulate proliferation and induce or delay differentiation. They stimulate other critical processes in cell function as well. So far, however, the molecular mechanisms of action of the FGF's are unknown. Nevertheless, so many new and varied functions have

---

Abbreviations: PA: plasminogen activator, aFGF: acidic fibroblast growth factor, bFGF: basic fibroblast growth factor, kb: kilobase, TGF_B: transforming growth factor, CSF: colony stimulating factor, EGF: epidermal growth factor, kD: kilodaltons, ECM: extracellular matrix, PA: plasminogen activator.

now been described for FGF's that, at present, one must consider these peptides to be of special importance for the control of cell growth and differentiation.

PRIMARY STRUCTURE, GENOMIC ORGANIZATION, AND mRNA EXPRESSION OF ACIDIC AND BASIC FGF

Basic FGF has been purified from most mesoderm- or neuroectoderm- derived tissues or cells which have in common a strong angiogenic potential (Table 1, Gospodarowicz, 1986a; 1986b). Structural studies have shown that bFGF is a single chain peptide composed of 146 amino acids (Esch et al., 1985a) which can also exist in an NH_2-terminally truncated form missing the first 15 amino acids (Gospodarowicz et al., 1985). The truncated form of bFGF is as potent as native bFGF, as demonstrated by radioreceptor binding and biological assays, indicating that the NH_2-terminal region of bFGF is neither involved in its binding to FGF cell surface receptors nor in its biological activity (Neufeld and Gospodarowicz, 1986). Related to bFGF is aFGF, which shares a 55% total sequence homology with bFGF (Esch et al., 1985b). Acidic FGF is a 140-amino acid peptide which can also exist as an NH_2-terminally truncated form missing the first 6 amino acids: des. 1-6 aFGF (Gimenez-Gallego et al., 1986). The high degree of homology between aFGF and bFGF suggests that they are derived from a common ancestral gene.

Evidence that a viral oncogene may code for a growth factor or part of a growth factor receptor has recently emerged from studies on the PDGF structure and on the

Table 1. *Normal and neoplastic tissues or normal and transformed cells containing bFGF*[a]

Normal or transformed tissue	Cultured normal diploid cells	Cultured tumor cells
Brain	Corneal endothelial cells	Y-1 Adrenal cortex cells
Retina	Capillary endothelial cells	Osteosarcoma U2OS
Pituitary	Pituitary cells	Ewing's sarcoma
Kidney	Ovarian granulosa cells	Rhabdomyosarcoma
Placenta	Adrenal cortex cells	Melanoma
Corpus Luteum	Lens epithelial cells	Hepatoma (Sk HP-1)
Adrenal Glands	Uterine epithelial cells	Retinoblastoma
Immune System	Myoblasts	
(Macrophage-Monocyte)	Retinal pigmented epithelial cells	
Prostate	Vascular smooth muscle cells	
Bone	Astrocytes	
	Osteoblasts	
Cartilage		
Chondrosarcoma		
Melanoma		

[a] So far, aFGF has only been detected in brain, retina, bone matrix, osteosarcoma osteoblasts, astrocytes, and fetal vascular smooth muscle cells.

EGF receptor structure (Sporn and Roberts, 1985). In the case of basic FGF, a 46% and 42.3% homology, respectively, has been shown to exist with the predicted product of Int-2 and the hst gene product (Dickson and Peter, 1987; Taira et al., 1987). A lesser degree of structural homology exists between those two gene products and aFGF. While Int-2 has been implicated in the induction of virally induced mammary cancer (Dickson et al., 1984), the hst gene was originally identified as a transforming gene in DNA's from human stomach cancer (Sakamoto et al., 1986).

Basic FGF seems to have been extremely well conserved through evolution. For example, bovine and human bFGF differ in only 2 of their 146 amino acids, giving an overall amino acid sequence homology of 98.7% (Abraham et al., 1986b). Avian and bovine bFGF have the same amino acid composition and avian bFGF cross-reacts on an equimolar basis with bovine bFGF in an RIA using rabbit anti-bFGF polyclonal antibodies. Thus, homologous epitopes are well conserved (Gospodarowicz et al., 1987). Acidic FGF seems to be less well conserved, and the bovine form differs from the human by 11 amino acids out of a total of 146 (Abraham et al., 1987).

The FGF genes have been cloned and complementary DNA sequences of both bFGF and aFGF have been synthesized. The genomic organization of the genes encoding bFGF and aFGF has been described (Abraham et al., 1986a; 1986b; Mergia et al., 1987; Fig. 1). The bFGF gene is localized on human chromosome 4, while that of

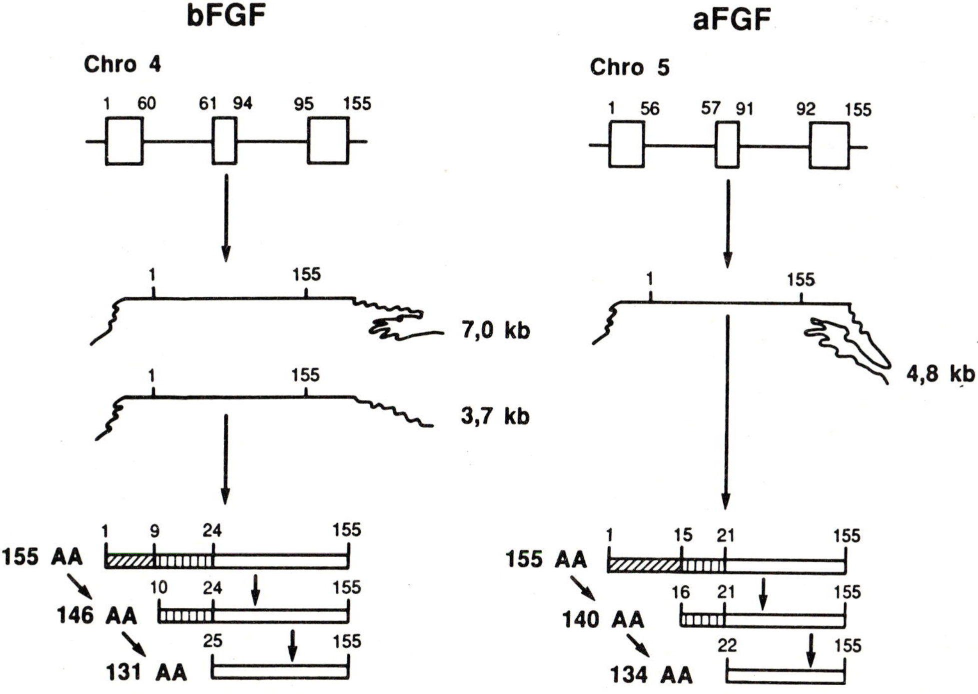

Figure 1. Genomic organization, mRNA transcripts, and cellular processing of bFGF and aFGF.

aFGF is on chromosome 5 (Abraham et al., 1987). This suggests that through a process of gene duplication and evolutionary divergence, bFGF and aFGF have become separate gene products. The basic FGF gene, with its size greater than 38 kbp, encodes three exons widely separated by two introns: the first one separates codons 60 and 61, and the second separates codons 94 and 95. The aFGF gene has a similar organization, with 2 large introns located in identical positions in the coding sequence once basic and aFGF are properly aligned (Fig. 1). Southern blot analysis of human genomic DNA has shown that there is only one bFGF and one aFGF gene. Therefore, all of the characterized or uncharacterized heparin binding endothelial cell mitogens related to bFGF or aFGF are the products of a single bFGF or aFGF gene (Abraham et al., 1986a; 1987). In various cultured cells and tissues, the bFGF gene gives rise to two polyadenylated mRNA's of approximately 3.7 and 7.0 kb (Gospodarowicz et al., 1987). The aFGF gene appears to encode a single mRNA species of approximately 4.1 kb (Jaye et al., 1986). The primary translation product for either bFGF or aFGF is composed of 155 amino acids. Proteolytic cleavage from the precursor molecule of the first 9 (bFGF) or 15 residues (aFGF) would result in the generation of the mature proteins which can then be cleaved further in homologous positions to give the NH_2-truncated form of bFGF (des. 1-15) or a FGF (des. 1-6) (Abraham et al., 1987; Gospodarowicz, 1987) (Fig. 1).

bFGF GENE EXPRESSION IN CELL TYPES WHICH DO NOT EXPRESS THE bFGF GENE, BUT RESPOND TO bFGF, RESULT IN AUTONOMOUS CELL PROLIFERATION

The concept of autocrine stimulation of cell proliferation postulates that a normal diploid cells can gain growth autonomy by acquiring the ability to produce, secrete, and respond to a given growth factor (Todaro et al., 1977; Sporn and Todaro, 1980). Verification of the autocrine hypothesis, in the case of bFGF, requires the demonstration that expression of an introduced FGF gene in non-tumorigenic cells results in or contributes to the malignant transformation of those cells.

The hypothesis that inappropriate expression of bFGF could lead to cell transformation has been tested by introducing into BHK-21 cells a plasmid that directs the high level expression of human bFGF. BHK-21 cells were chosen because they do not express the bFGF gene and, in previous studies, they have been shown to be totally dependent on exogenous bFGF in order to proliferate when maintained under serum-free conditions (Neufeld et al., 1986). Finally, exogenous bFGF induces anchorage-independent soft agar growth of BHK-21 cells. This effect, however, is transient, and cells revert to their normal phenotype once the mitogen is removed. High level bFGF expression in BHK-21 cells might therefore be expected to lead to permanent anchorage-independent soft agar growth of BHK-21 cells.

Southern blot analysis demonstrates that in BHK-21 cells, following transfection, at least one complete bFGF gene copy per cell has been stably incorporated; a second, partial copy also appears to be present. That the integrated foreign bFGF genes are actively expressed is indicated by the detection through Northern blot analysis of 0.6 and 4.3 kb RNA transcripts, which were not seen in the parental BHK-21 cell RNA, and which differed in size from those found in bovine, mouse, or human cells expressing the endogenous bFGF gene (3.7 and 7.0 kb, respectively). Additionally, transfected cells contained 6×10^6 bFGF molecules per cell, while no detectable bioactive FGF was found in the parental BHK-21 cells (Neufeld et al., 1988).

The drastic effect of high level expression of bFGF on the proliferation of cells which do not normally express the bFGF gene was evident from the cell behavior following transfection. BHK-21 cells, which, on solid substrate, have an absolute requirement for exogenous FGF in order to proliferate in serum-free medium, proliferated actively in the absence of exogenous bFGF once transfected with plasmids carrying the human bFGF coding sequence under the control of the SV40 enhancer and human metallothionein II_A promoter. Likewise, in soft agar, transfected cells formed colonies, while parental cells required the addition of exogenous bFGF in order to do so. This therefore demonstrates that whether bFGF interacts with its receptor within the cells, or at a surface location, it is capable of triggering the autonomous growth of a single cell in which it is synthesized in high amounts (Neufeld et al., 1988).

EXPRESSION OF bFGF AND aFGF IN TISSUES AND CULTURED CELLS

Organs/Tissues

So far, basic FGF has been purified from a wide variety of mesoderm- and neuroectoderm-derived organs and tumors (Table 1) (Gospodarowicz et al., 1986a; 1986b). Depending on the organ from which bFGF is isolated, the predominant forms are either the 146 or 131 amino acid long forms, with smaller amounts of the 155 amino acid long form being present. It is not known whether these various forms coexist in the tissues, or if they are artefactually created by specific proteases during FGF extraction and isolation (Ueno et al., 1986). The 140 and 136 amino acid truncated aFGF forms are the predominant molecular species, with a small amount of the 155 amino acid-long form present. So far, aFGF has only been found in brain, retina, bone matrix, osteosarcoma (Gospodarowicz et al., 1986a; 1986b) and various gliomas (Liberman, 1987). Since aFGF is 30- to 100-fold less potent than bFGF, it contributes to only 8% and 0.15% respectively of the total mitogenic activity present in crude brain or retinal extract, with the rest contributed by bFGF (Gospodarowicz et al., 1986b).

Cultured Cells

All organs that contain bFGF are heavily vascularized. This suggested that cells of the vascular system might synthesize bFGF. In fact, vascular endothelial cells express the bFGF gene, and they synthesize bioactive bFGF (Schweigerer et al., 1987a). In contrast, they do not express the aFGF gene or bioactive aFGF. Thus, bFGF could act as an autocrine growth factor for vascular endothelial cells. The synthesis of bFGF in vascular endothelial cells also provides an explanation for the rather ubiquitous distribution of bFGF. Basic FGF is also expressed in a wide variety of other normal

58

diploid cells, all of which are sensitive to bFGF in vitro (Gospodarowicz et al., 1986b; 1987) (Table 1). Various tumors derived from those cells also express bFGF (Table 1). This has led to the proposal that uncontrolled expression of bFGF could be involved in the development and in the progression of tumors (Schweigerer et al., 1987b; Gospodarowicz et al., 1987).

The demonstration of the presence of bFGF in various normal diploid or tumor cells has also provided clues for its possible function in the most unexpected locations. For example, it has recently been reported that mineralized matrix of osseous tissue harbors abundant mitogenic activity, represented in part by bFGF and aFGF (Hauschka et al., 1986b). The cellular sources of FGF present in bone matrix had not been defined. However, the demonstration of bFGF in cultured osteoblast (Gospodarowicz et al., 1987) suggests that bFGF could be produced by that cell type in vivo, and that it could act in an autocrine or paracrine manner. Basic FGF is also produced in cells derived from retinoblastoma (Gospodarowicz et al., 1987), a tumor thought to be derived from photoreceptor cells. Thus, it is possible that photoreceptors are the source of bFGF within the normal retina.

Although this localization of bFGF would not be predictable based on what was previously known of its biological activity, it has recently been demonstrated that bFGF is a component of the rod's outer segment, where it is strongly bound to rhodopsin (Plouet et al., 1986). This suggests a possible role of bFGF in phototransduction. Finally, the localization of bFGF in cell types which have no function yet assigned to them provides new insights on their possible physiological functions. Pituitary glands are known to contain high concentrations of bFGF (Gospodarowicz, 1974), but the cell types responsible for synthesis of pituitary bFGF were unknown. Recent studies have shown that the main cellular source of bFGF in pituitary are follicular cells which can contain as many as 5×10^5 bFGF molecules per cell (Ferrara et al., 1987). Previous studies (Gon et al., 1987) have suggested that follicular cells may play an important role in the restoration of degenerated pituitary glandular tissues during the early stage of transplantation. This is in agreement with the suggestion by Farquhar et al. (1975) that follicular cells play the role of nurse cells in the pituitary gland, similar to that of the Sertoli cells in the testes. Follicular cells are also involved in extracellular matrix (ECM) synthesis (Vila-Porcile and Oliver, 1985), and there is a large amount of experimental evidence that indicates that ECM plays an important role in cell growth and differentiation (Gospodarowicz et al., 1982).

Previous studies have shown that FGF controls the production of ECM components and could become an integral part of such structures (see "FGF and the extra cellular matrix"), thereby further supporting the growth and differentiation of cells becoming associated with newly produced ECM. The ability of follicular cells to support the restoration of pituitary granular cells could therefore reflect their ability to synthesize and release FGF associated with ECM components, such as heparan sulfate proteoglycans. It has also been suggested that follicular cells, which are mainly concentrated in the pars tuberalis, would provide support for the portal vessels. The presence of an angiogenic factor such as bFGF in follicular cells could therefore relate to the development and maintenance of the differentiated state of the pars tuberalis microvasculature.

THE FGF RECEPTORS

All cell types which respond to bFGF or aFGF bear specific FGF cell surface receptors. In the baby hamster kidney (BHK-21) cell line, the density of FGF cell surface receptors is 10- to 30-fold higher than that of normal diploid cells. In BHK-21 cells, bFGF binds to specific high-affinity cell surface receptors ($k_d = 0.27$ nM; 1.2×10^5 binding sites per cell). This compares with a k^d for aFGF of 0.25 nM and 8.7×10^4 binding sites per BHK-21 cell. As expected from the high degree of structural homology between bFGF and aFGF, both mitogens bind to the same receptor. Basic FGF and aFGF do not bind to other growth factor receptors, nor do other growth factors bind to the FGF receptor (Gospodarowicz et al., 1986a; 1986b). Cross-linking of bFGF or aFGF to the BHK-21 cell surface receptor indicates that qualitatively, both mitogens interact with the same two M_r 145 kD and 125 kD membrane components, which could differ by their degree of glycosylation. Quantitatively, bFGF appears to display a higher affinity than aFGF for the $M_r = 145$ kD receptor species, while aFGF displays a higher affinity than bFGF for the $M_r = 125$ kD receptor species (Neufeld and Gospodarowicz, 1986). This could help in explaining the different biological potencies of bFGF versus aFGF (see below).

The FGF receptors of muscle cells, Swiss 3T3 fibroblasts, lens epithelial cells, human umbilical vein endothelial cells, rhabdomyosarcoma, Ewing's sarcoma (SK-ES1), and PC-12 cells have also been characterized (Table 2). They all share similar molecular weight ranges, but might differ by their degree of glycosylation. However, in all cases both bFGF and aFGF interact with the same receptor, with k_d's ranging from 45 pM to 200 pM (Table 2) (Gospodarowicz et al., 1987).

Table 2. *Characterization of FGF receptors on various cell types*

Cell types	MW(kD)	k_d	Receptors/cells
Muscle cells	165[ab]	11pM[ab]	2×10^3[ab]
Swiss 3T3	160[ab]	45pM[ab]	6×10^4[ab]
Murine capillary endothelial cells	150 and 130[a]	ND	ND
Human umbillical endothelial cells	130[ab]	ND	ND
PC-12	145[ab]	20pM[ab]	3.6×10^3[ab]
Rhabdomyosarcoma	125 and 145[ab]	ND	ND
SK-ES1 cells	150[b]	76pM[b]	1.4×10^4[b]
BHK-21 cells	125 and 145[ab]	270pM[ab]	1×10^5[ab]
Lens epithelial cells	145	53pM[b]	2×10^4[b]

ND = not determined
 a = determined with aFGF
 b = determined with bFGF
ab = determined with both basic and acidic FGF.

IN VITRO BIOLOGICAL EFFECT OF FGF

Most of the biological studies with FGF have been done with the basic form. Only recently has the biological activity of aFGF started to be investigated. As expected from its high degree of structural homology with bFGF, aFGF has a mitogenic effect identical to that of bFGF, although it is, depending on the cell type, 30- to 100-fold less potent (Gospodarowicz, 1986a; 1986b). The lower potency of aFGF makes it a weak agonist of the basic form, and may reflect the qualitatively different interactions of aFGF versus bFGF with its cell surface receptor species (Gospodarowicz et al., 1986a; 1986b). Basic FGF has both acute and long-term effects on the morphology and growth pattern of responsive cells. It increases their migratory activity (Gospodarowicz, 1985), and it makes confluent cultures of BALB/c 3T3 cells look "transformed" in that it induces reduced cell-substratum adhesion, growth in crisscross pattern, and increased membrane ruffling (Gospodarowicz and Moran, 1974). Basic FGF can also induce the growth in soft agar of non-transformed cells, and in that model it potentiates the effect of TGF_B (Gospodarowicz et al., 1986b).

Basic FGF is a potent mitogen for mesoderm-derived cells (Gospodarowicz, 1987) (Table 3), triggering cell proliferation with half-maximal and maximal effects at 1.5 and 10 pM, respectively. Basic FGF is mitogenic both for cells seeded at clonal density and for low-density cultures (Gospodarowicz, 1979), and greatly reduces their average cellular doubling time. This is primarily due to a shortening of the G1 phase of the cell cycle (Gospodarowicz et al., 1978).

Basic FGF stabilizes the phenotypic expression of cultured cells (Table 3) (Gospodarowicz, 1985). This property is particularly interesting, since it has made possible the long-term culturing of cell types that otherwise would lose their normal phenotype in culture when passaged repeatedly at low cell density (Gospodarowicz et al., 1978). This biological effect of bFGF has been studied exhaustively in endothelial cells derived from large vascular vessels or cornea that were cloned and maintained in the presence of bFGF and then deprived of it for various time periods (Gospodarowicz et al., 1979; Gospodarowicz, 1985; 1987). This effect of bFGF on cell differentiation may be due to its ability to control the synthesis and deposition of various basement membrane/ECM components that are know to affect cell surface polarity and gene expression. These include collagen, fibronectin, laminin, and proteoglycans (Gospodarowicz and Greenburg, 1981; Gospodarowicz, 1983). Basic FGF can also induce capillary endothelial cells to invade a three-dimensional collagen matrix and to organize themselves to form characteristic tubules that resemble blood capillaries. Concomitantly, bFGF stimulates endothelial cells to produce a urokinase-type plasminogen activator (PA), a protease that has been implicated in the neovascular response. Thus bFGF can stimulate processes that are characteristic of angiogenesis in vivo, including endothelial cell migration, invasion, and production of plasminogen activator (Montesano et al., 1986).

When added to chondrocytes (Kato and Gospodarowicz, 1985), bFGF can act as a mitogen as well as a differentiating agent. While costal chondrocytes grown in absence of bFGF soon assume a fibroblastic appearance and lose their ability to synthesize and release chondroitin sulfate, proteoglycans, and collagen type II, cells grown in the presence of bFGF retain these capabilities and at confluence become embedded in a

Table 3. *Cell types for which basic or acidic FGF is mitogenic or affects differentiation*

Normal diploid cells	Basic FGF	Acidic FGF
Glial and astroglial cells	+(D)	+
Oligodendrocytes	+(D)	+
Trabecular meshwork cells	+	?
Endothelial cells from capillary, large vessel and endocardium	+(D)	+(D)
Corneal endothelial cells	+(D)	+(D)
Fibroblasts	+	+
Myoblasts	+(D)	+(D)
Vascular smooth muscle	+	+
Chondrocytes	+(D)	+(D)
Osteoblasts	+	+
Blastema cells	+	?
Adrenal cortex cells	+	+
Granulosa cells	+	+
Prostatic epithelial cells	+	+
Mesothelial cells	+	+
Neuronal cells	+	?
Established cell lines		
Rat fibroblast-1	+	+
Balb/c 3T3	+	+
Swiss 3T3	+	+
BHK-21	+	+
A-204 rhabdomyosarcoma	+	?
PC-12	(D)	(D)

(D) = induces differentiation
+   = positive effect on cell proliferation
?   = effect on cell proliferation not determined

thick ECM which has all of the characteristics of that produced in vivo (Kato and Gospodarowicz, 1985). Interestingly enough, cells will express their correct phenotype only if exposed to bFGF when dividing actively; when added to confluent layers of dedifferentiated and resting chondrocytes, bFGF can no longer reverse their phenotype. bFGF also has a pronounced effect on astrocytes, stimulating both their proliferation and the differentiation as reflected by its positive effect on the synthesis of glial fibrillary acidic protein (Pettman et al., 1985; Morrison et al., 1985).

Probably the most spectacular effect of bFGF on cell differentiation is observed with nerve cells. Togari and co-workers (1983; 1985) first reported that bFGF acts as a differentiation factor in a rat pheochromocytoma (PC-12) cell line by inducing both neurite outgrowth and ornithine decarboxylase activity. Later it was shown that aFGF has similar properties (Neufeld et al., 1987; Wagner and D'Amore, 1986), and that PC-12 cells express specific FGF receptor sites. Similar effects of bFGF on nerve cells have been reported by Walicke et al. (1986), using highly purified populations of fetal rat hippocampal neurons. Under well-defined serum-free cell culture conditions, bFGF can increase both neuronal survival and neurite extensions. Furthermore, the addition of bFGF to rat cerebral cortical neurons markedly enhances their survival and the elaboration of neurites (Morrison et al., 1986). These results suggest that bFGF may function as a neurotropic agent in the central nervous system.

Not all of the effects of bFGF on cell differentiation are positive effects. For example, bFGF can delay differentiation and fusion of myoblasts (Gospodarowicz et al., 1976). In some established myoblast cell lines, bFGF and aFGF can induce a decrease in creatine phosphokinase expression (Lathrop et al., 1985a). These inhibitory FGF effects on differentiation have been attributed to the ability of FGF to keep myoblast populations in an active proliferative stage, thereby decreasing the percentage of cells in slow growing populations which would enter during their extended G_0, G_1 phase into a stage of terminal differentiation (Lathrop et al., 1985b).

AGENTS MODULATING THE BIOACTIVITY OF FGF

Heparin is one of the factors that can modulate the bioactivity of FGF. It potentiates the mitogenic activity of aFGF on BHK-21 or human umbilical endothelial cells by a hundred-fold, thus rendering it as potent as bFGF. In PC-12 cells, heparin has similar effects on the neurotropic activity of aFGF (Gospodarowicz et al., 1987).

It has been proposed that in vivo heparin could affect aFGF in much the same fashion as those effects reported in vitro. However, an assumption of complete correspondence may be misleading: all studies treating the potentiation of heparin/aFGF bioactivity have, to date, been performed using highly purified aFGF, which may have lost much of its own intrinsic bioactivity (normally exhibited in vivo) following acid treatment and other harsh protocols of the purification process (Gospodarowicz and Cheng, 1986; Gimenez-Gallego et al., 1986). Therefore, when released by cells in vivo, and in its native state, aFGF could be as potent as bFGF.

Protamine sulfate can also modify the biological response to FGF. Protamine sulfate can act as an inhibitor of angiogenesis in vivo, and it markedly inhibits the ability of bFGF or aFGF to stimulate the proliferation of vascular endothelial cells in vitro (Neufeld and Gospodarowicz, 1987). The inhibition is reversible and the cells remain viable even after prolonged exposure to protamine sulfate. Protamine sulfate inhibits the mitogenic effects of both growth factors by preventing their interaction with FGF cell surface receptors (Gospodarowicz et al., 1987). In contrast, protamine sulfate potentiates the mitogenic activity of EGF; this indicates that it can also act at cellular sites which are not associated with FGF receptors (Neufeld and Gospodarowicz, 1987).

TGF_B, depending on the cell type upon which FGF acts, can either potentiate or inhibit its activity while having no activity of its own. This reflects the multifunctional properties of TGF_B which has been shown to both stimulate or inhibit cell proliferation or differentiation (Sporn et al., 1986). TGF_B strongly potentiates the mitogenic activity of bFGF on osteoblasts (Globus and Gospodarowicz, 1987). In contrast, TGF_B inhibits the mitogenic activity of bFGF and aFGF on vascular endothelial cells (Baird and Durkin, 1986; Frater-Schroder et al., 1986). The ability of TGF_B to inhibit the activation of PA as well as the release of other proteases, which are positively regulated by bFGF and which may be crucial for ECM degradation during angiogenesis, may be relevant to some of its inhibitory effects on vascular endothelial cell proliferation triggered by FGF. Since TGF_B and FGF can interact at the cellular level to modulate growth, it suggests that many of the biological activities of FGF observed in vitro and in vivo may be regulated by the presence of TGF_B and related proteins in the local cellular milieu.

FGF AND THE EXTRACELLULAR MATRIX

In the early stage of embryonic development, the different tissues composing an organ are formed as a result of strictly timed and spatially interrelated proliferative and differentiative events. This involves the interaction of cells with newly formed ECM, a process that promotes their proliferation and which stabilizes their newly acquired phenotype (Gospodarowicz et al., 1982). ECM components have been implicated in inductive tissue interaction, somite chondrogenesis, differentiation of corneal epithelium, salivary gland morphogenesis, tooth germ development, and nephron formation (Gospodarowicz, 1985). Previous studies have shown that ECM produced by vascular or corneal endothelial cells can mimic all of the effects of bFGF, including those on cell proliferation and/or differentiation (Gospodarowicz and Tauber, 1980; Gospodarowicz and Greenberg, 1981; Gospodarowicz et al., 1982). Serum or plasma-derived growth factors, purified ECM components such as fibronectin, laminin, or various collagen types are not responsible for these effects, suggesting that FGF associated with ECM components might be the active factor. Indeed, bFGF has a high affinity for heparin. This glycosaminoglycan is closely related to heparn sulfate, which is produced in large quantities by both corneal and vascular endothelial cells, and is a structural component of their ECM (Gospodarowicz et al., 1987). The possibility therefore exists that FGF could be secreted by the cells in association with extracellular matrix components and become an integral part of the ECM.

Indirect evidence for the integration of bFGF into an insoluble substrate such as the ECM can also be derived from the observation that media conditioned by capillary or corneal endothelial cells has no significant impact on their proliferation. In contrast, their own denuded ECM will induce them to rapidly proliferate and assume the proper phenotype once confluent. Thus bFGF, in contrast to other conventional growth factors such as TGF_B, EGF, and PDGF, may not be released in a soluble form (Gospodarowicz et al., 1986a; 1986b). This is in agreement with the fact that neither bFGF nor aFGF are synthesized with a conventional signal peptide (Abrahams et al., 1986; Jay et al., 1986). Both growth factors, however, might be associated with ECM components, and as such, be transported to the cell exterior, where they could interact with specific FGF cell surface receptors to induce their biological effects (Vlodavsky et al., 1987), or be stored in the ECM and later released following hydrolysis of ECM components. In that context, it is interesting to note that during morphogenesis of lobular organs, the areas with the greatest mitotic activity are located in areas where hydrolysis of the ECM occurs. Similarly, in the kidney, angiogenesis correlates well with the hydrolysis of the kidney mesenchymal stroma. In the adult, heparan sulfate present in ECM could be degraded by heparitinase, an enzyme released either by platelets, when they attach to the subendothelium, or by macrophages once they are activated (Gospodarowicz et al., 1986b). This could ultimately lead to the solubilization of heparan sulfate/FGF complexes which would be biologically active, and could participate in various repair or developmental processes.

OTHER REGULATORY FUNCTIONS OF FGF

As in the case of EGF, which is known to modulate the synthesis and release of prolactin and growth hormone by GH3 cells, bFGF can increase the release of prolactin and decrease the basal level of growth hormone secreted by Ch_4C_1 cells (Gospodarowicz et al., 1986b) or primary cultures of rat anterior pituitary cells (Baird et al., 1986).

In rat granulosa cells, which do not respond to bFGF by an increase in proliferative rate, bFGF inhibits the FSH-mediated induction of the LH receptor and reversibly attenuates the FSH-induced cell aromatase activity. This tends to suggest that FGF may play an inhibitory cytodifferentiative role in the ontogeny of the granulosa cells (Baird et al., 1986; Gospodarowicz et al., 1987).

The positive correlation of plasminogen activator (PA) expression and the proliferation of solid tumors point to an instrumental role for this enzyme in neoplastic growth, a role that is likely to involve the degradation of matrix and basement membrane proteins by plasmin or plasmin-activated proteases. It has been shown that bFGF could increase PA production in certain mammary carcinoma cells without inducing their replication in vitro. Among the factors which could influence PA expression induced by bFGF is TGF_B. This growth factor has been shown to inhibit the production of secreted proteases in response to bFGF and increase the production of a PA inhibitor (Nilsen-Hamilton et al., 1987).

IN VIVO EFFECTS OF FGF

In early embryonic development, the basic body plan arises because cells in different regions of the egg become programmed to follow different pathways (Slack, 1983). During oogenesis, differences arise between the animal and vegetal halves of the eggs. Fertilization results in a subdivision of the vegetal half into a dorsal-vegetal and a ventro-vegetal region. Mesoderm is then induced from the animal hemisphere by signal(s) originating from the vegetal region of the egg (Nieuwkoop, 1969; Slack, 1983). This induction is an instructive phenomenon that suppresses epidermal differentiation of cells from the animal pole, and directs them instead to differentiate into mesodermal cells. Signal(s) originating from the dorsal-vegetal region lead to the formation of dorsal-type mesoderm, mostly consisting of notochord and somites, while signal(s) originating from the ventro-vegetal region lead to the formation of ventral-type mesoderm, consisting primarily of blood cells, mesenchyme, and mesothelium.

In recent studies Slack and his colleagues (1987) have investigated the possibility of bFGF mimicking the effect of the ventro-vegetal signal(s) responsible for the formation of ventral-type mesoderm. Tissue explants isolated from animal pole of stage 8 Xenopus blastulae normally differentiate into epidermis or undifferentiated epidermal cells. When similar explants are exposed to bFGF, cells differentiated instead into mesodermal structures. Between 2 to 30 ng bFGF/ml, the induction closely resembled ventral-type mesoderms formed by explants where ventrovegetal regions were combined with animal poles. They consisted of concentric arrangements of loose mesenchyme, mesothelium, and blood cells within an epidermal jacket. At higher bFGF concentrations (30 to 120 ng/ml) most of the explants contained significant amounts of muscle blocks (Slack et al., 1987). The inducing effect of bFGF seems to be highly specific, since it could not be mimicked by other growth factors such as TGF_B or $TGF\alpha$, TNF Interferons α and γ, insulin, Interleukin-1α and β, G-CSF and GM-CSF (colony-stimulating factors).

Therefore, in early embryo, bFGF can act as a primordial differentiation factor, inducing the ectoderm to become mesoderm. This is in close agreement with previous in vitro studies which have shown that FGF had a transforming activity and could act as a morphogen, as well as a mitogen, on practically all mesoderm-derived cells studied to date. The FGF capability to induce mesoderm formation in early embryo is also of interest in view of its partial structural homology with the oncogene Int-2 (Dickson and Peters, 1987). This oncogene has been reported to be present only prior to day 7.5 of gestation in the mouse, and is most abundantly expressed in cells of the primitive endodermal lineage (Jakobovits et al., 1986).

In lower vertebrates (amphibians) bFGF can promote limb regeneration (Gospodarowicz and Mescher, 1981). This tends to support the concept that bFGF could be involved in the neurotropic control of this process (Gospodarowicz et al., 1986b). In addition to being a neurotrophic factor involved in limb regeneration, bFGF could also play a role in the early development of the nervous system. Basic FGF promotes both the survival and differentiation of nerve cells derived either from the hippocampus or the neocortex. Nerve cells have also been shown to contain bFGF (Pettman et al., 1986), and preliminary studies have demonstrated that neuronal cell populations derived from early embryonic brain do proliferate in response to bFGF, and later express cholinergic differentiation. All these effects point towards bFGF's possible role in CNS development. FGF could also have pronounced effects on the proliferation and differentiation of other brain cell populations, such as astrocytes and oligodendrocytes, by influencing their glial properties during normal development or subsequent to a specific pathogenic event (Gospodarowicz et al., 1987). Through its angiogenic properties bFGF could influence CNS development, since it has been reported that FGF could be responsible for capillary ingrowth into the brain (Risau, 1986).

Basic FGF, which has been detected in macrophages, could play a crucial role in the wound healing processes, following its release from the damaged cells. Interestingly, bFGF, unlike other growth factors such as EGF, PDGF or TGF_B, can stimulate both in vitro as well as in vivo the proliferation of all the cell types involved in wound healing (Gospodarowicz et al., 1986a; 1986b). These include capillary endothelial cells, vascular smooth muscle, and fibroblasts, notwithstanding other cell types which are involved in the wound healing of specialized territories, such as chondrocytes, myoblasts, etc. (Gospodarowicz, 1979; 1985). Basic FGF also increases the formation of granulation tissue in vivo (Gospodarowicz, 1985), and the synthetic function of fibroblasts and

66

myoblasts. It also stimulates the rate of reepithelialization of the epidermis detached from dermis after blister induction. In other tissues such as cartilage bFGF can promote chondrossification, and its presence in bone matrix could indicate that it could play an important role in the development and growth of osseous tissue (Gospodarowicz et al., 1987).

Basic FGF acts as a potent angiogenic factor in vivo, as demonstrated by the rabbit cornea, the chick chorioallantoic membrane (CAM) or the hamster cheek pouch assays. These observations are supported by the demonstration of bFGF as the major angiogenic agent in richly vascularized tissues such as corpus luteum, adrenal gland, kidney, and retina (Gospodarowicz et al., 1986 a; 1986b; Baird et al., 1986).

Recent studies have shown that bFGF is identical to the tumor angiogenic factor (Klagsbrun et al., 1986). Thus, bFGF might play an important role in tumor progression. By increasing capillary endothelial cell proliferation, and inducing the sprouting of new capillaries into solid tumors, bFGF might allow an increased O_2 and nutrients supply to tumor cells and also facilitate metastasis. Basic FGF could also act at the level of the tumor cell itself. By increasing its PA level as well as by increasing the secreted levels of various proteases and collagenase, bFGF would facilitate the metastasic process and tumor invasion (Gospodarowicz et al., 1987). It could also act as a mitogen for the tumor cells. The normal diploid cells listed in Table 3 are either uniquely dependent on bFGF or they require various growth factors including FGF, EGF, and PDGF in order to proliferate (Gospodarowicz et al., 1978). Upon neoplastic transformation of cells that depend only on FGF, uncontrolled expression of bFGF in these cells could occur and make them divide in an uncontrolled manner. In the case of cells responding to multiple growth factors, uncontrolled expression of bFGF might make them independent of other exogenous growth factors during their growth phase.

CONCLUSION

The importance of FGF in the ontogeny of development and biopathology of mesenchymal tissues can no longer be ignored. The recent molecular characterization of FGF as well as the cloning and mapping of its genes, has led to the general consensus that all the numerous heparin-binding growth factors were, in fact, represented by 2 single gene products: basic and acidic FGF. The further demonstration that both basic and acidic FGF have a high degree of structural homology and bind to the same receptor has led to the conclusion that they had identical biological roles, although they differed in their specific activity.

Probably one of the most important questions to be resolved is the in vivo role of FGF. The high degree of structural conservation of bFGF through species as different as mammalian, avian and amphibian, as well as its presence in all vertebrates studied to date — including piscean — indicate that in vivo FGF could have a very primordial role. This is, in fact, what seems to be indicated by the studies of Slack et al. (1987), which have shown that bFGF can act as a primordial morphogen at one of the earliest embryonic stages, inducing the transformation of cells destined to be ectodermal, into mesenchymal cells. This is consistent with the in vitro properties of bFGF, which has been shown to act as mitogen as well as morphogen for mesenchymal cells studied to date. It is also in agreement with the ability of bFGF to support the regeneration proces in lower vertebrates.

One of the most popularized aspects of the in vivo biology of FGF is based on its angiogenic activity. Basic FGF has been shown to induce in early embryo the appearance of blood islands and its effects on capillary endothelial cells in vitro or in vivo, as well as its distribution in various organs or tumors known to have angiogenic potential, provide a common denominator for its widespread angiogenic activity. However, narrowing the experimental focus to FGF's angiogenic properties would produce an extremely limited view of its potential targets in vivo. The cell types listed in Table III clearly indicate in which organ an effect of FGF, either in tissue formation or repair process, should be investigated. In particular, the in vivo mitogenic and differentiation effects of bFGF on various cell types of the nervous system would be worth investigating, since it has been shown to control both the proliferation and differentiation of oligodendrocytes, and astrocytes, as well as acting as a triggering mechanism for the differentiation of nerve cells in vitro.

Although it is likely that bFGF could still control the proliferation and differentiation of mesenchymal cells later in the ontogeny of development, little is actually known about the implication of the activation of the FGF gene expression in neoplastic transformation. It has been speculated that activation of growth factor-controlling gene expressed early in embryogenesis and later repressed could lead to neoplastic transformation (Sporn and Roberts, 1985). Transfection of normal diploid cells such as vascular endothelial cells with plasmids carrying FGF-cDNA, resulting in the constitutive expression of bFGF, could be a useful approach to testing that hypothesis. Cells expressing high bFGF levels could also be used for studies dealing with the locus of action of FGF (either intra- or extracellular locations), the transcellular transport of FGF and pathways of FGF release from the cells. Of equal importance will be studies dealing with mechanisms and factors controlling the expression of the FGF receptor, since this process would ultimately determine the time, as well as the cell type, which would be FGF-responsive. Such studies cannot be initiated until we have a better understanding of the molecular properties of the FGF receptor, and in particular, until we have cloned FGF receptor cDNA, which can later be used to study its expression.

REFERENCES

Abraham A, Whang L, Tumolo A, Mergia A, Fiddes JC (1987) Human basic fibroblast growth factor: nucleotide sequence genomic organization and expression in mammalian cells. In: Molecular Biology of Homo Sapiens, Vol. 51. Cold Spring Harbor, New York, pp. 657-668.

Abraham JA, Whang JL, Tumolo A, Mergia A, Friedman J, Gospodarowicz D, Fiddes JC (1986a) Human basic fibroblast growth factor: nucleotide sequence and genomic organization. EMBO (Europ Molec Biol Org) J 5:2523-2528.

Abraham JA, Mergia A, Whang JL, Tumolo A, Friedman J, Hjerrild KA, Gospodarowicz D, Fiddes JC (1986b) Nucleotide sequence of a bovine clone encoding the angiogenic protein, basic fibroblast growth factor. Science, Washington D.C. 233:545-548.

Baird A, Durkin T (1986) Inhibition of endothelial cell proliferation by type B transforming growth factor: interactions with acidic and basic fibroblast factors. Biochem Biophys Res Commun 138:476-482.

Baird A, Esch F, Mormede P, Ueno N, Ling N, Böhlen P, Ying SY, Wehrenberg WB, Guillemin R (1986) Molecular characterization of fibroblast growth factor: distribution and biological activities in various tissues. Recent Prog in Hormone Research 42:143-205.

Dickson C, Peters G (1987) Potential oncogene product related to growth factors. Nature 326:833.

Dickson C, Smith R, Brookes S, Peters G (1984) Tumorogenesis by mouse mammary tumor virus: Proviral activation of a cellular gene in the common integration region Int-2. Cell 37:529-536.

Esch F, Baird A, Ling N, Ueno N, Hill F, Deneory R, Klepper R, Gospodarowicz D (1985a) Primary structure of bovine pituitary basic fibroblast growth factor (FGF) and comparison with the amino terminal sequence of bovine brain acidic FGF. Proc Natl Acad Sci USA 85:6507-6511.

Esch F, Ueno N, Baird A, Hill F, Denoroy L, Ling N, Gospodarowicz D, Guillemin R (1985b) Primary structure of bovine brain acidic fibroblast growth factor (FGF). Biochem Biophys Res Commun 133:554-562.

Farquhar MG, Stutelsky EH, Hopkins CR (1975) Structure and function of the anterior pituitary and dispersed pituitary cells. In Vitro Studies. In: A Tixer-Vidal, MG (eds): The Anterior Pituitary Gland. Farquhar, Academic Press, New York, pp. 82-135.

Ferrara N, Schweigerer L, Neufeld G, Gospodarowicz D (1987) Pituitary follicular cells produce basic fibroblast growth factor. Proc Natl Acad Sci USA 84:5773-5777.

Frater-Schroder M, Muller G, Burchmeier W, Böhlen P (1986) Transforming growth factor B inhibits endothelial cell proliferation. Biochem Biophys Res Commun 137:295-302.

Gimenez-Gallego G, Conn G, Hatcher VB, Thomas KA (1986) Human brain-derived acidic and basic fibroblast growth factors: amino terminal sequences and specific mitogenic activities. Biochem Biophys Res Commun 135:561-566.

Globus R, Gospodarowicz D (1987) Fibroblast growth factor is a mitogen for cultured osteoblasts. Endocrinology, submitted.

Gon G, Shirasawa N, Ishikawa H (1987) Appearance of the cyst or ductile like structures and their role in the restoration of the rat pituitary autograft. Anat Rec 217:371-378.

Gospodarowicz D (1974) Localization of a fibroblast growth factor and its effect alone and with hydrocortisone on 3T3 cell growth. Nature, London 249:123-127.

Gospodarowicz D (1979) Fibroblast and epidermal growth factors: their uses in vivo and in vitro in studies on cell functions and cell transplantation. Mol Cell Biochem 25:79-110.

Gospodarowicz D (1983) The control of mammalian cell proliferation by growth factors, extracellular matrix and lipoproteins. J Inv Derm 81:41-50.

Gospodarowicz D (1985) Biological activity in vivo and in vitro of pituitary and brain fibroblast growth factor. In: Ford RJ, Maizel AL (eds): Mediators in Cell Growth and Differentiation. Raven Press, New York, pp. 109-134.

Gospodarowicz D (1987) Purification of brain and pituitary FGF. In: Barnes D, Sirbasku D (eds): Methods in Enzymology: Peptide growth factors. Academic Press, Orlando, FL, 147:106-119.

Gospodarowicz D, Cheng J (1986) Heparin protects basic and acidic FGF from inactivation. J Cell Physiol 128:475-484.

Gospodarowicz D, Cheng J, Lui GM, Baird A, Esch F, Böhlen P (1985) Corpus luteum angiogenic factor is related to fibroblast growth factor. Endocrinology 117:2283-2291.

Gospodarowicz D, Cohen DC, Fujii DK (1982) Regulation of cell growth by the basal lamina and plasma factors: relevance to embryonic control of cell proliferation. In: Sato G, Pardee A, Sirbasku D (eds): Cold Spring Harbor Conferences on Cell Proliferation, vol. 9: Growth of cells in hormonally deficient media. Cold Spring Harbor, New York, pp. 95-124.

Gospodarowicz D, Greenburg G (1981) Growth control of mammalian cells. Growth factors and extracellular matrix. In: Ritzen M, Aperia A, Hall K, Larsson A, Zetterberg A, Zetterstrom R (eds): The Biology of Normal Human Growth. Raven Press, New York, pp. 1-21.

Gospodarowicz D, Greenburg G, Bialecki H (1978) Factors involved in the modulation of cell proliferation in vivo and in vitro: the role of fibroblast and epidermal growth factors in the proliferative response of mammalian cells. In Vitro 14:85-118.

Gospodarowicz D, Ferrara N, Schweigerer L, Neufeld G (1987) Structural characterization and biological functions of fibroblast growth factor. Endocrine Review 8:95-114.

Gospodarowicz D, Mescher Al (1981) Fibroblast growth factor and vertebrate regeneration. In: Riccardi VM, Mulvihill JJ (eds): Advances in Neurology: Neurofibromatosis, vol 29. Raven Press, New York, pp. 149-171.

Gospodarowicz D, Moran J (1974) Effect of a fibroblast growth factor, insulin, dexamethasone, and serum on the morphology of BALB/c 3T3 cells. Proc Natl Acad Sci USA 71:4648-4652.

Gospodarowicz D, Neufeld G, Schweigerer L (1986a) Fibroblast growth factor. Mol Cell Endocrin 46:187-206.

Gospodarowicz D, Neufeld G, Schweigerer L (1986b) Molecular and biological characterization of fibroblast growth factor: an angiogenic factor which also controls the proliferation and differentiation of mesoderm and neuroectoderm-derived cells. Cell Differ 19:1-17.

Gospodarowicz D, Tauber J-P (1980) Growth factors and extracellular matrix. Endocrine Review 1:201-227.

Gospodarowicz D, Vlodavsky I, Greenberg G, Alvarado J, Johnson LK, Moran J (1979) Cellular shape is determined by the extracellular matrix and is responsible for the control of cellular growth and function. In: Ross R, Saro G (eds): Cold Spring Harbor Conferences on Cell Proliferation, Vol 6: Hormones and Cell Culture. Cold Spring Harbor, New York, pp. 561-592.

Gospodarowicz D, Weseman J, Moran J (1975) Presence in the brain of a mitogenic agent distinct from fibroblast growth factor that promotes the proliferation of myoblasts in low density culture. Nature, London 256:216-220.

Gospodarowicz D, Weseman J, Moran J, Lindstrom J (1976) Effect of fibroblast growth factor on the division and fusion of bovine myoblast. J Cell Biol 70: 395-405.

Hauschka PV, Mavrakas AE, Iafrati MD, Doleman SE, Klagsbrun N (1986) Growth factors in bone matrix: isolation of multiple types by affinity chromatography on heparin-Sepharose. J Biol Chem 261:12665-12674.

Jaye M, Howk R, Burgess W, Ricca GA, Chiu IM, Ravera MW, O'Brien SJ, Modi WS, Maciag T, Drohan WN (1986) Human endothelial cell growth factor: cloning, nucleotide sequence, and chromosome localization. Science. 233: 541-544.

Jakobovits A, Shackleford GM, Varmus HE, Martin GR (1986) Two proto-oncogenes implicated in mammary carcinogenesis, Int-1 and Int-2, are independently regulated during mouse development. Proc Natl Acad Sci USA 83:7806-7810.

Kato Y, Gospodarowicz D (1985) Sulfated proteoglycan synthesis by rabbit costal chondrocytes grown in the presence and absence of fibroblast growth factor. J Cell Biol 100:477.

Klagsbrun M, Sasse J, Sullivan R, Smith JA (1986) Human tumor cells synthesize an endothelial cell growth factor that is structurally related to basic fibroblast growth factor. Proc Natl Acad Sci USA 83:2448-2452.

Lathrop B, Olson E, Glaser L (1985a) Control by fibroblast growth factor of differentiation in the BC3H1 muscle cell line. J Cell Biol 100:1540-1548.

Lathrop B, Olson E, Glaser L (1985b) Control of myogenic differentiation by fibroblast growth factor is mediated by position in the G1 phase of the cell cycle. J Cell Biol 101:2194-2202.

Liberman TA, Friesel R, Jaye M, Lyall RM, Westermark B, Drohan W, Schmidt A, Maciag T, Schlessinger J (1987) An angiogenic growth factor is expressed in human glioma cells. EMBO J 6:1627-1632.

Mergia A, Tumolo A, Haaparanta T, Whang JL, Gospodarowicz D, Abraham JA, Fiddes JC (1987) Isolation and characterization of the human gene for acidic FGF, in preparation.

Montesano R, Vassali JD, Baird A, Guillemin R, Orci L (1986) Basic fibroblast growth factor induces angiogenesis in vitro. Proc Natl Acad Sci Usa 83:7297-7301.

Morrison R, DeVeillis J, Lee YL, Bradshaw RA, Eng LF (1985) Hormones and growth factors induced the synthesis of glial fibrillary acidic protein in rat brain astrocytes. J Neurosci Res 14:167-172.

Morrison RS, Sharma A, DeVeillis J, Bradshaw A (1986) Basic fibroblast growth factor supports the survival of cerebral cortical neurons in primary culture. Proc Natl Acad Sci USA 83:7537-7541.

Neufeld G, Gospodarowicz D, Dodge L, Fujii DK (1986) Heparin modulation of the neurotropic effects of acidic and basic fibroblast growth factors and nerve growth factors on PC-12. J Cell Physiol 131:131-140.

Neufeld G, Gospodarowicz D (1987) Basic acidic fibroblast growth factor interact with the same cell surface receptor. J Biol Chem 261:5631-5637.

Neufeld G, Gospodarowicz D (1987) Protamine sulfate inhibits the mitogenic activities of the extracellular matrix and FGF, but potentiates that of epidermal growth factor. J Cell Physiol 132:287-294.

Neufeld G, Massoglia S, Gospodarowicz D (1986) Effect of lipoproteins and growth factors on the proliferation of BHK-21 cells in serum-free cultures. Regulatory Peptides 13:293-305.

Neufeld G, Ponte P, Mitchell R, Gospodarowicz D (1988) Expression of human basic fibroblast growth factor cDNA in baby hamster kidney-derived cells results in autonomous cell growth. J Cell Biol, April.

Nieuwkoop P (1969) The formation of mesoderm in Urodelean amphibians. I. Induction by the endoderm. Wilhelm Roux' Arch Entw Mech Org 162:341-373.

Nilsen-Hamilton M, Hamilton RT (1987) Detection of proteins induced by growth regulators. Methods in Enzymology 147:427-444.

Pettman B, Labourdette G, Weibel M, Sensenbrenner M (1986) The brain fibroblast growth factor (FGF) is localized in neurons. Neurosci Letters 68:175-179.

Pettman B, Weibel M, Sensenbrenner M, Labourdette G (1985) Purification of two astroglial growth factors from bovine brain. FEBS Letters 189:102-108.

Plouet J, Mascarelli F, Lagente O, Dorey C, Lorans G, Faure J.-P, Courtois Y (1986) Eye derived growth factor: a component of rod outer sement implicated in phototransduction. In: Agardh E, Ehinger B (eds): Retinal Signal Systems, Degenerations and Transplants. Elsevier Science Publishers BV, New York, pp. 311-320.

Risau W (1986) Developing brain produces an angiogenesis factor. Proc Natl Acad Sci USA 83:3855-3859.

Sakamoto H, Mori M, Taira M, Yoshida T, Matsukawa S, Shimizu K, Sekiguchi M, Terada M, Sugimura T (1986) Transforming gene from human stomach cancers and a non-cancerous portion of stomach mucosa. Proc Natl Acad Sci USA 83:3997-4001.

Schweigerer L, Neufeld G, Friedman J, Abraham JA, Fiddes JC, Gospodarowicz D (1987a) Capillary endothelial cells express basic fibroblast growth factor, a mitogen that stimulates their own growth. Nature, London 325:257-259.

Schweigerer L, Neufeld G, Mergia A, Abraham JA, Fiddes JC, Gospodarowicz D (1987b) Basic fibroblast growth factor in human rhabdomyosarcoma cells: implications for the proliferation and neovascularization of myoblast-derived tumors. Proc Natl Acad Sci USA 84:842-846.

Slack JM (1983) From egg to embryo: determinative events in early development. Cambridge University Press, Cambridge and London.

Slack JM, Darlington B, Heath H, Godsave S (1987) Heparin binding growth factors as agents of mesoderm induction in early Xenopus embryo. Nature 326:197-200.

Sporn MB, Roberts AB (1985) Autocrine growth factor and cancer. Nature 313:745-747.

Sporn MB, Roberts AB, Wakefield LM, Assoian RK (1986) Transforming growth factor$_B$: biological function and chemical structure. Science 233:532-534.

Sporn MB, Todaro GJ (1980) Autocrine secretion malignant transformation of cells. N Eng J Med 303:878-880.

Taira M, Yoshida T, Miyagawa K, Sakamoto H, Terada M, Sugimura T (1987) cDNA sequence of human transforming gene hst and identification of the coding sequence required for transforming activities. Proc Natl Acad Sci USA 84:2980-2984.

Todaro GJ, DeLarco E, Nissley SP, Rechler MM (1977) MSA and EGF receptors on sarcoma virus-transformed cells and human fibrosarcoma cells in culture. Nature, London 267:526-528.

Togari A, Baker D, Dickens G, Guroff G (1983) The neurite-promoting effect of fibroblast growth factor on PC-12 cells. Biochem Biophys Res Commun 144:1189-1196.

Togari A, Dickens G, Huzuya J, Guroff G (1985) The effect of fibroblast growth factor on PC-12 cells. J Neurosci 5:307-315.

Ueno K, Baird A, Esch F, Ling N, Guillemin R (1986) Isolation of an amino acid terminal extended form of basic fibroblast growth factor. Biochem Biophys Res Commun 138:580-588.

Vila-Porcile E, Olivier L (1984) The problem of the folliculo-stellate cells in the pituitary gland. In: PM Motta (ed): Ultrastructure of Endocrine Cells and Tissues. Martinus Nijhoff Publishers, Boston, pp. 64-76.

Vlodavsky I, Folkman J, Sullivan R, Frieman R, Ishai R, Michaeli Sasse J, Klagsbrun M (1987) Endothelial cell-derived basic fibroblast growth factor: Synthesis and deposition into subendothelial extracellular matrix. Proc. Natl Acad Sci USA 84:2282-2296.

Wagner JA, D'Amore P (1986) Neurite outgrowth induced by an endothelial cell mitogen isolated from retina. J Cell Biol 103:1363-1370.

Walicke P, Cowarn M, Ueno K, Baird A, Guillemin R (1986) Fibroblast growth factor promotes survival of dissociated hippocampal neurons and enhances neurite extension. Proc Natl Acad Sci USA 83:3012.

Neuronal Plasticity and Trophic Factors
G. Biggio, P.F. Spano, G. Toffano, S.H. Appel, G.L. Gessa (eds.)
Fidia Research Series, Symposia in Neuroscience VII
Liviana Press, Padova © 1988

8-SUBSTITUTED cAMP ANALOGS CAN REPLACE THE NGF REQUIREMENT OF CULTURED RAT SYMPATHETIC AND SENSORY NEURONS: EVIDENCE FOR PARALLEL NEUROTROPHIC PATHWAYS

Russell E. Rydel and Lloyd A. Greene

Department of Pharmacology, New York University School of Medicine,
550 First Avenue, New York, NY 10016, USA

INTRODUCTION

The development, maintenance and repair of neurons are regulated at least in part via specific neurotrophic factors. Characterization of these factors and of their molecular mechanisms is important since this will not only provide a basic understanding of neuronal behavior, but has the potential to lead to amelioration of conditions resulting from injury, degeneration or maldevelopment of the nervous system. Given such potential major practical applications of neurotrophic factors, it will also be important to find means to mimic or enhance their activities.

At present, the best characterized neurotrophic agent is the nerve growth factor (NGF) (Levi-Montalcini and Angeletti, 1968; Greene and Shooter, 1980; Thoenen and Edgar, 1985). NGF exerts its actions on sympathetic, sensory and certain CNS neurons. The precise molecular mechanisms of NGF action have yet to be fully described. One aspect of the NGF mechanism that has been extensively studied is the role of cAMP therein (cf. Greene and Shooter, 1980; Richter-Landsberg and Jastorff, 1986, for review). At present, the bulk of evidence suggests that cAMP is not the second messenger for NGF action. It is, however, not conclusively clear whether or not cAMP represents at least a necessary component of the NGF mechanism.

Present address: Laboratory of Cellular and Molecular Neurobiology, Department of Pathology, Columbia University College of Physicians and Surgeons, New York, NY 10032.

We describe here studies in which dissociated cell cultures of rat neonatal sympathetic and embryonic dorsal root ganglionic neurons were used to screen a variety of agents for their ability to mimic the neurotrophic actions of NGF. In particular, recent findings (Rydel and Greene, 1987) are reviewed and amplified which provide evidence that certain, but not all, membrane permeant analogs of cAMP can promote the survival of these two neuronal types as well as stimulate them to produce neurites. We further review and supplement evidence that the neurotrophic activities of NGF and of these cAMP derivatives are mediated by different molecular mechanisms. These findings have several practical implications which will be addressed in the discussion.

RESULTS

Effect of Various Agents on Survival of Cultured Rat Neonatal Sympathetic Neurons

Although NGF has been established to be the principal neurotrophic factor responsible for maintenance of sympathetic neurons both in vivo and in vitro, a variety of agents were tested for their capacities to replace or mimic NGF in culture. Accordingly, postnatal day 1-3 rat superior cervical ganglion cells were dissociated and plated on collagen- or laminin-coated culture dishes as previously described (Rydel and Greene, 1987) in a medium containing 85% RPMI 1640 medium, 10% horse serum, 5% fetal bovine serum, and the presence or absence of various additives. In some cases, 10 μM cytosine arabinoside was included from the first to seventh day after plating to kill and suppress the growth of non-neuronal cells. The agents tested were chosen because of their known effects either on other types of neurons or on PC12 rat pheochromocytoma cells (Greene and Tischler, 1982).

In the absence of additives, less than 10% of the neurons plated survive even for 24 hr (Fig. 1A). In contrast, when NGF is included in the medium at a concentration of 2 nM, nearly all plated neurons survive at 24 hr (Fig. 1B), and about 60-70% survive by a week after plating. With NGF present, the neurons also produce an extensive network of neurites (Fig. 2 B,D). Of the various agents tested, 8-Br cGMP or dibutyryl cGMP (0.01-2 mM), basic fibroblast growth factor (300 pM), insulin (200 nM), elevated K$^+$ (45 mM) and a phorbol ester (12-0-tetradacanoylphorbol 13-acetate; 4 nM-1 μM) each failed to maintain neuronal survival (Rydel and Greene, 1987). The lack of effect of these drugs was not due to a direct toxic action since none had an evident negative influence on NGF-promoted survival or neurite outgrowth.

The one class of agents tested that was fully effective in replacing NGF comprised 8-substituted membrane-permeant analogs of cAMP (Rydel and Greene, 1987). Two derivatives, 8 (4-chlorophenylthio) cAMP (CPT-cAMP; optimal dose 0.3-1 mM) and 8-Br cAMP (optimal dose 1-3 mM) were found to promote neuronal survival to a similar extent as NGF, even after at least one month in culture. Moreover, the neurons also extended neurites and the density of this neuritic network continued to increase over time of treatment (Figs. 1 and 2). The actions of these cAMP analogs appear to be directly on the neurons since their neurotrophic effects were not altered by elimination of essentially all the non-neuronal cells in the cultures by exposure to cytosine arabinoside.

In contrast to the C8-substituted derivatives, several N^6-substituted cAMP analogs were only partially effective in replacing NGF (Rydel and Greene, 1987). After 1 week of treatment, N^6, $O^{2'}$-dibutyryl cAMP (optimal concentration 0.3-1 mM) and N^6, $O^{2'}$-dioctanoyl cAMP (optimal concentration 0.1-0.3 mM) maintained about 30% of the number of neurons that NGF maintained. Similar results were achieved with forskolin (optimal concentration 3-100 μM), an activator of adenylate cyclase. The relative ineffectiveness of these derivatives was not caused by their having any direct toxic activities since they did not interfere with (nor did they enhance) NGF-promoted sympathetic neuron survival or process outgrowth.

Further experiments were carried out to test whether the C8-substituted cAMP derivatives were in fact addressing the same population of sympathetic neurons as NGF (Rydel and Greene, 1987). Neuronal cultures were established with either NGF or CPT-cAMP present. After one week, the cultures were extensively washed and the types of treatment exchanged. Thus, neurons initially maintained with NGF were exposed to CPT-cAMP and *vice versa*. In each case, the numbers of neurons in the cultures at various times after the switch were comparable to those in control cultures in which the types of treatments were not exchanged. Such findings led to the conclusion that NGF and CPT-cAMP exert their neurotrophic actions on the same populations of sympathetic neurons. In agreement with this, provision of optimal doses of both NGF and CPT-cAMP together does not lead to greater numbers of surviving neurons than obtained with either agent alone (Fig. 1).

The Neurotrophic Actions of NGF and C8-Substituted cAMP Analogs Take Place Via Different Pathways

Although both NGF and C8-substituted cAMP analogs promote sympathetic neuron survival and process outgrowth, their effects can be distinguished (Rydel and Greene, 1987). First, on a collagen substrate, appreciable numbers of neurites do not appear in the CPT- or 8Br- cAMP-treated cultures for the first several days after plating (Fig. 1C). In contrast, with NGF, most of the neurons bear neurites within the first day of plating (Fig. 1B). Second, even after longer periods of treatment, the density of outgrowth in the cultures exposed to the cAMP analogs is less extensive than in cultures maintained with NGF (Fig. 2). This is true for both collagen (Figs. 1; 2 A,B; 3 A,B) and laminin (Fig. 2 C,D) as substrates. Third, NGF produces a marked hypertrophy of the neuronal cell bodies while the cAMP derivatives do not (Fig. 2). These differences do not appear to be due to any negative effect of CPT- or 8Br- cAMP since cultures containing both NGF and the analogs are similar in appearance to those maintained with NGF alone (Fig. 1).

Another indication of the difference between the pathways utilized by NGF and the cAMP analogs is their differential sensitivity to adenosine 3', 5'-phosphorothioate (Rp-cAMPS), a competitive cAMP antagonist (Rothermel et al., 1983; 1984; Richter-Landsberg and Jastorff, 1986). After 4 days of treatment, Rp-cAMPS almost completely blocked the ability of CPT-cAMP to maintain sympathetic neuron survival (Fig. 3, compare panels B and D; Rydel and Greene, 1987). In contrast, this inhibitor had little or no effect on NGF-promoted survival or neurite outgrowth (Fig. 3, compare

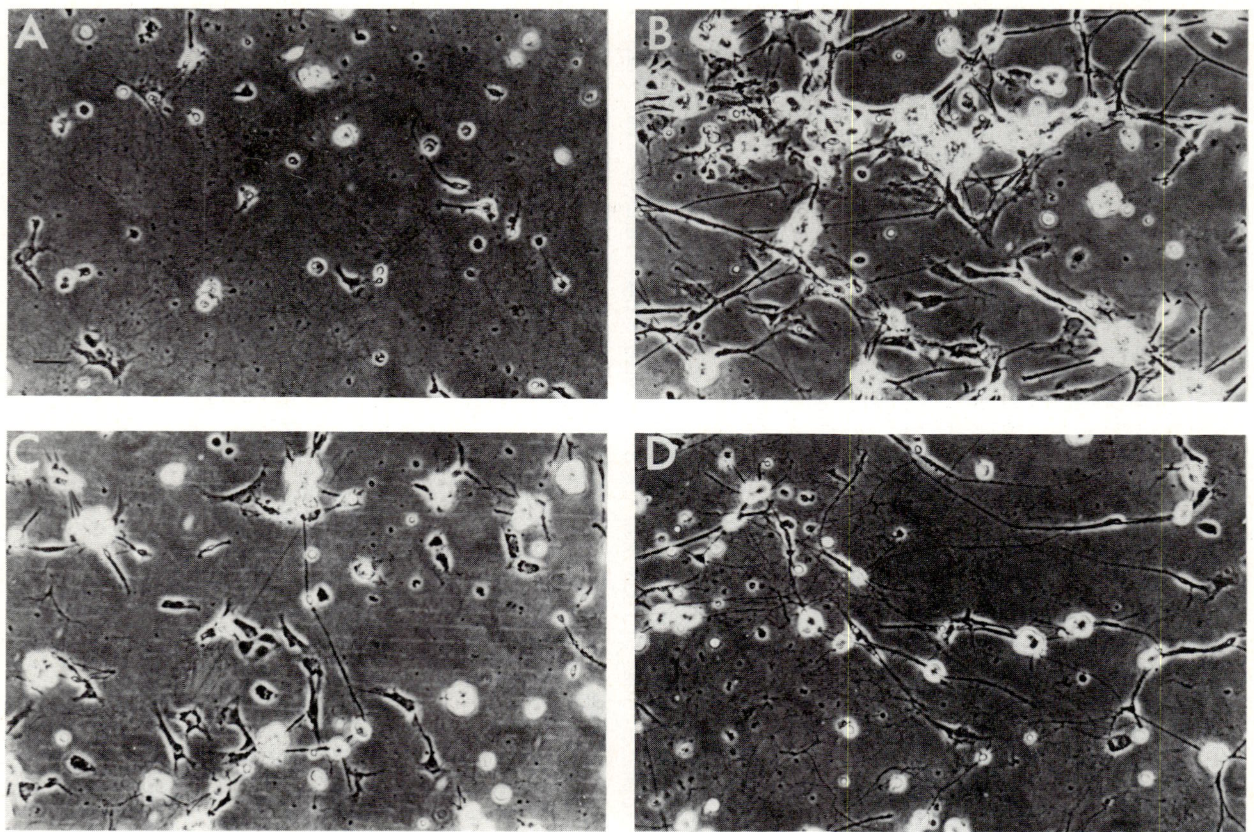

Figure 1. Comparison of the short-term effects of NGF and CPT-cAMP on sympathetic neuron survival and morphology. Phase contrast micrographs of newborn rat sympathetic ganglion cells 1 day after plating on a collagen substrate in the presence of either: A, medium without NGF; B, 50 ng/ml NGF; C, 0.3 mM CPT-cAMP; D, NGF+CPT-cAMP. Bar represents 50 μm.

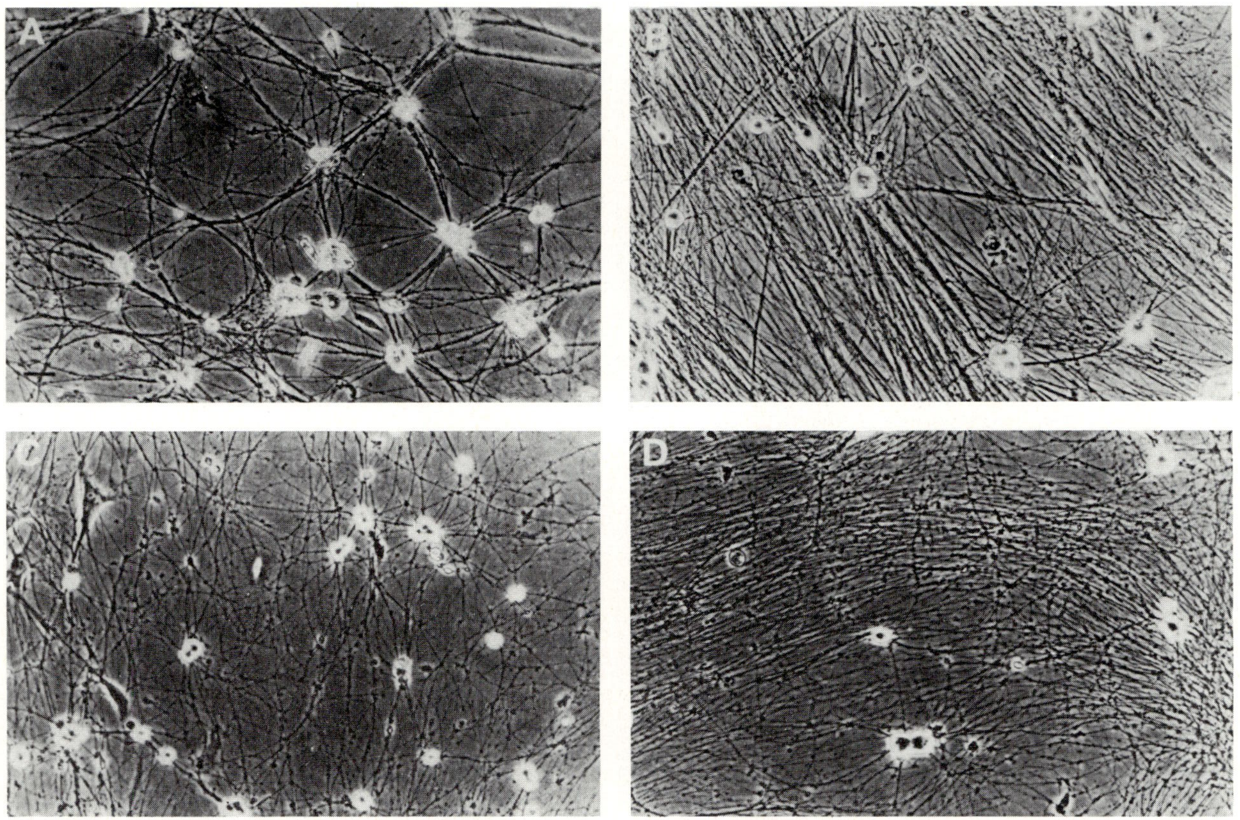

Figure 2. Comparison of the long-term effects of NGF and CPT-cAMP on sympathetic neuron survival and morphology. Phase contrast micrographs of newborn rat sympathetic ganglion cells 8 days after plating. A, Collagen substrate, 0.3 mM CPT-cAMP; B, Collagen substrate, 50 ng/ml NGF; C, Laminin substrate, 0.3 mM CPT-cAMP; D, Laminin substrate, 50 ng/ml NGF. Bar represents 50 μm.

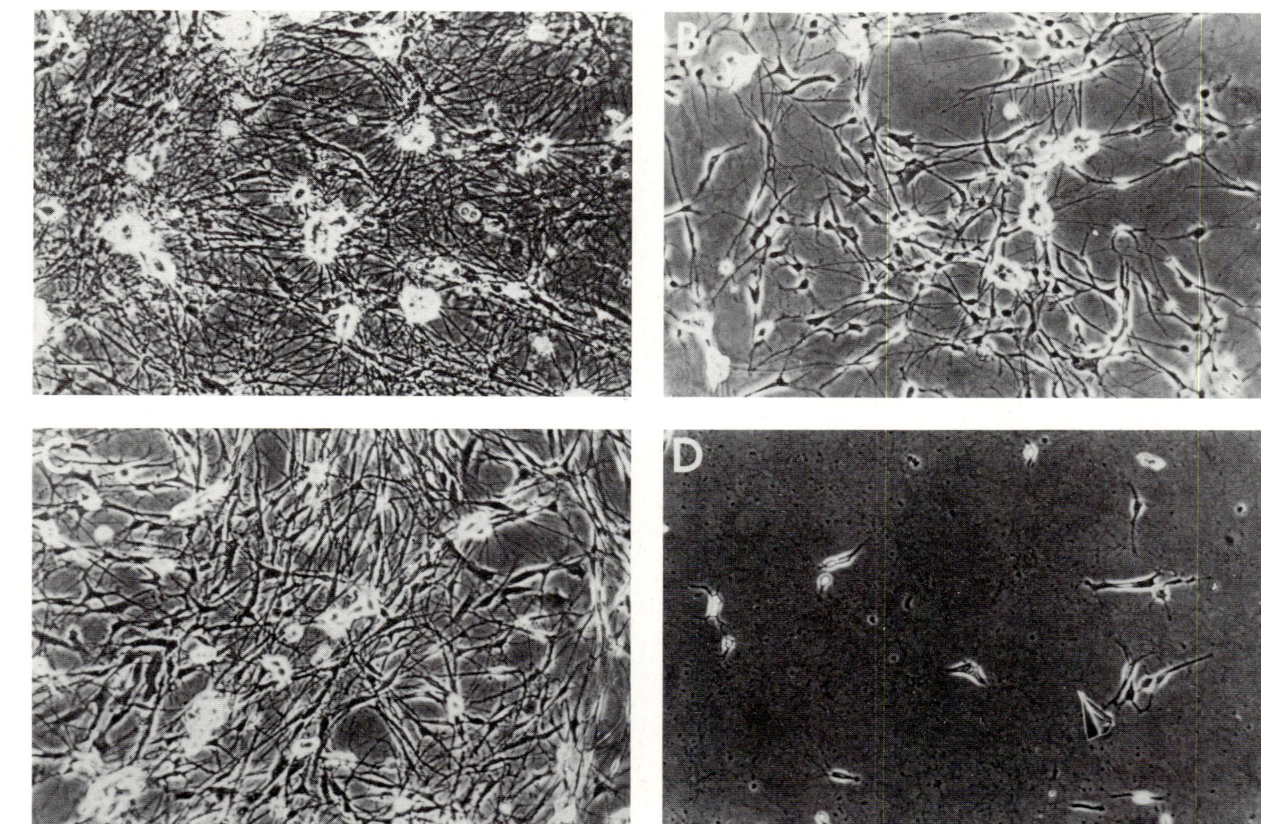

Figure 3. Comparison of the effects of the cAMP antagonist Rp-cAMPS on the neurotrophic activities of NGF and CPT-cAMP in sympathetic neuron cultures. Phase contrast micrographs of newborn rat sympathetic ganglion cells cultured on a collagen substrate for 4 days in the presence of either: A, NGF; B, CPT-cAMP; C, NGF + Rp-cAMPS; D, CPT-cAMP + Rp-cAMPS. Bar represents 50 μm.

panels A and C; Rydel and Greene, 1987). These observations indicate that the neurotrophic actions of the C8-substituted cAMP derivatives are mediated via a cAMP-dependent pathway. The most likely target would appear to be cAMP-activated protein kinase(s). These findings are also consistent with a number of others that appear to preclude a role for cAMP as a second messenger in the NGF mechanism (Greene and Shooter, 1980; Richter-Landsberg and Jastorff, 1986). Moreover, the ability of NGF to promote apparently normal responses in the presence of Rp-cAMPS further suggests that cAMP-dependent pathways are *not required* for the action of NGF.

Neurotrophic Actions of CPT-cAMP on Cultured Embryonic Rat Dorsal Root Sensory Neurons

To test whether CPT-cAMP could exert neurotrophic activities on another NGF-responsive target, experiments were also carried out with cultured embryonic rat dorsal root ganglia. Sensory ganglia were dissected from 15-day-old rat embryos, dissociated and plated at a density of 8-11 ganglia in 35 mm culture dishes as previously described (Rydel and Greene, 1987) in medium containing 15% fetal bovine serum. Under these conditions the sensory neurons require NGF for at least the first 5 days in vitro (Figs. 4 and 5). As with sympathetic neurons, CPT-cAMP is able to support sensory neuron survival in these cultures. Over the first 24-48 hr, similar numbers of neurons are present in both the NGF- and CPT-cAMP-treated cultures (Rydel and Greene, 1987). By 5 days of treatment, CPT-cAMP continues to maintain the neurons (Fig. 4), but preliminary cell counts indicate that there is some loss of numbers relative to cultures maintained with NGF (Fig. 5A). Such observations could indicate some heterogeneity of the population with respect to their responsiveness to cAMP analogs. By about 10 days of culture, the sensory neurons no longer show deterioration when either NGF or CPT-cAMP are removed and thus, as previously noted, are no longer dependent on extrinsically-provided neurotrophic support.

In addition to supporting survival, CPT-cAMP also promotes neurite outgrowth in the sensory neuron cultures (Fig. 4). However, as compared with neurons cultured for comparable periods with NGF, the neurons in the analog-treated cultures have a lesser-developed neurite network (Fig. 4). Also, the CPT-cAMP-treated sensory neurons do not show the somatic hypertrophy that occurs with NGF (Fig. 4). These differences were not due to any negative effect of the analog since neurons maintained with both NGF and CPT-cAMP exhibited neuritic densities and somatic hypertrophies characteristic of neurons treated with NGF alone (Fig. 4B, C, D). These differences in morphology suggest that NGF and the cAMP analogs affect sensory neurons via different mechanistic pathways.

Several observations indicate that, as in the case of sympathetic neurons, CPT-cAMP affects the same population of sensory neurons that respond to NGF. Co-treatment with NGF and the cAMP derivative does not enhance the number of neurons that survive for 24-48 hr in vitro. Also, after 5 days, the number of neurons surviving with a combination of the two treatments is no greater than that with NGF alone (Fig. 5A). Yet another indication is provided by a "switching" experiment. Sensory neurons cultures were maintained for 5 days in the presence of both NGF and

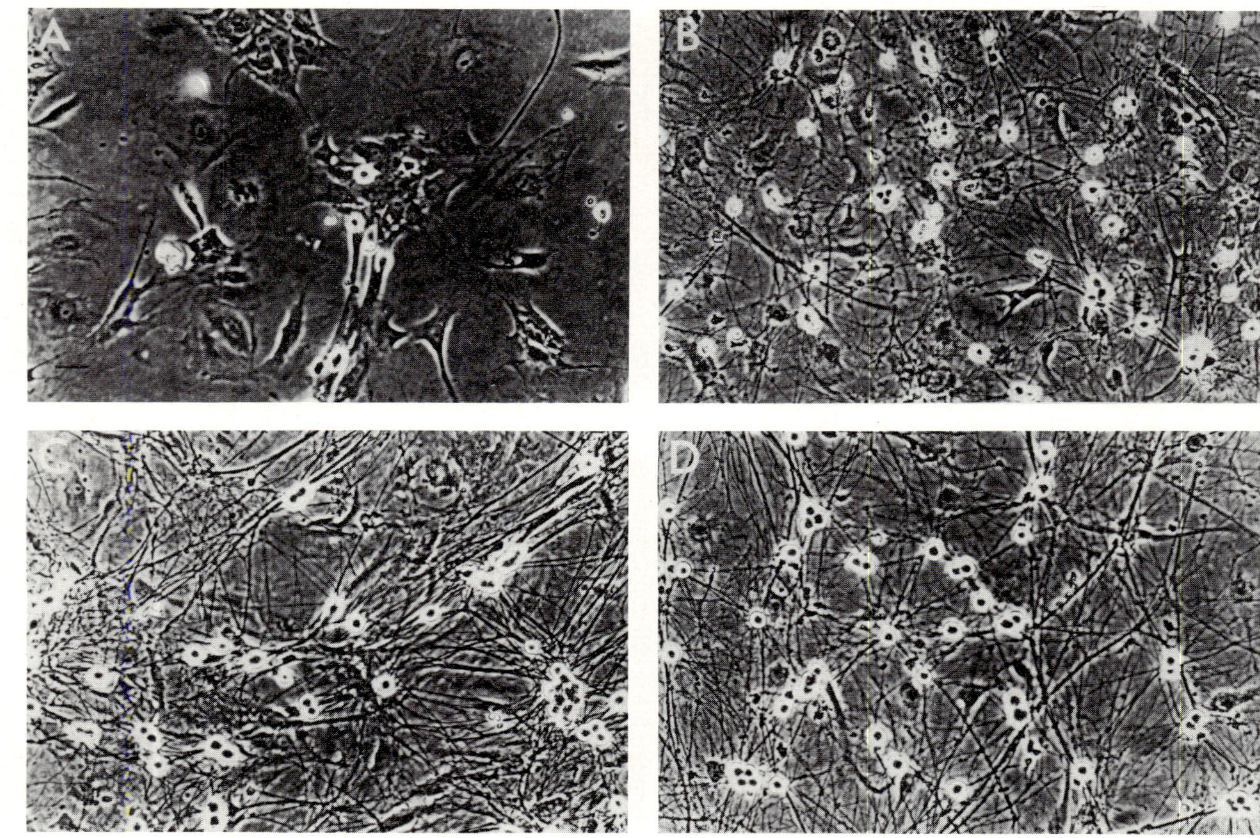

Figure 4. Comparison of the effects of NGF and CPT-cAMP on the survival and morphology of embryonic rat dorsal root ganglion cells. Phase contrast micrographs of cells cultured for 5 days on a laminin substrate in the presence of: A, medium without NGF or CPT-cAMP; B, 0.3 mM CPT-cAMP; C, NGF; D, NGF + 0.3 mM CPT-cAMP. Bar represents 50 μm.

CPT-cAMP and then cultured for an additional 5 days with either NGF+CPT-cAMP, NGF, CPT-cAMP, or no additive (control). Whereas removal of both agents caused most of the neurons to die, removal of either one of the agents had little or no effect on neuronal numbers (Fig. 5B).

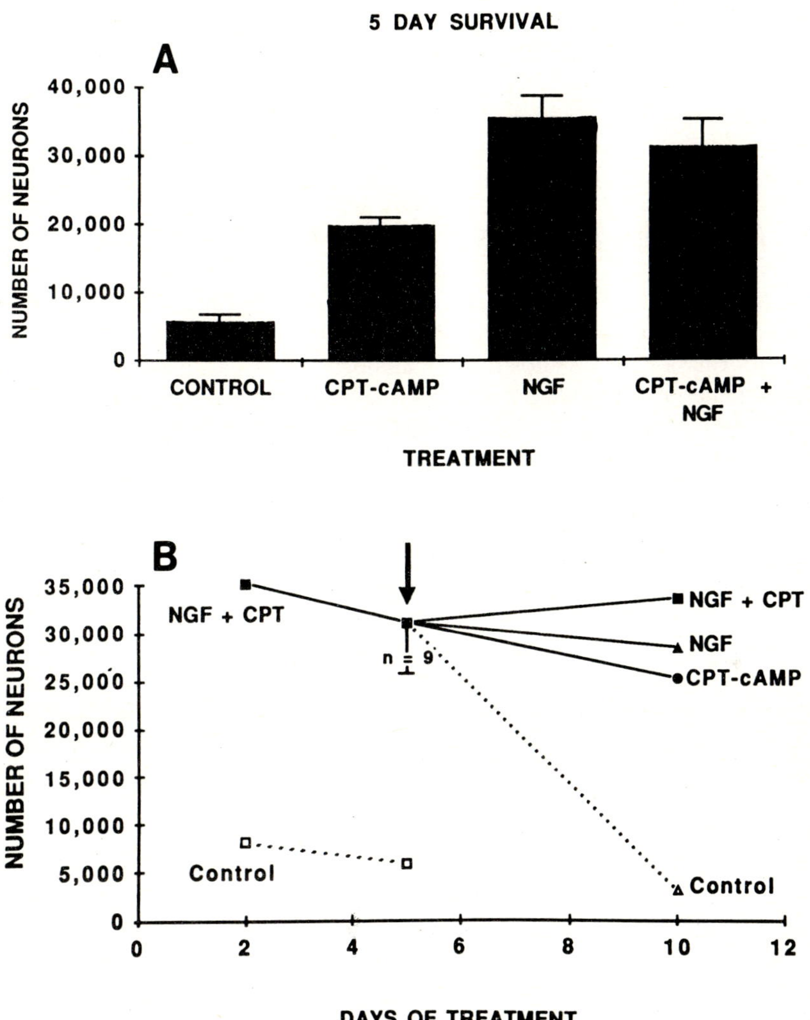

Figure 5. A. The effects of NGF and CPT-cAMP on the survival of embryonic rat dorsal root ganglionic neurons after 5 days in culture. Control represents cultures maintained without NGF or CPT-cAMP. Cell counts were performed as described elsewhere (Rydel and Greene, 1987) on sister cultures maintained under the indicated conditions. B. Evidence that CPT-cAMP and NGF affect the same populations of dorsal root ganglionic neurons. Embryonic rat dorsal root ganglionic cells were cultured for 5 days in the presence of both NGF and CPT-cAMP. The cultures were then washed extensively and cultured for an additional 5 days under the indicated conditions.

DISCUSSION

The aim of this paper has been to present evidence that C8-substituted cAMP derivatives can exert neurotrophic actions on mammalian sympathetic and DRG neurons. In particular, these derivatives can support the survival and differentiation of the same population of these neurons as NGF. Furthermore, our findings indicate that NGF and 8-substituted cAMP analogs elicit their neurotrophic actions via distinct primary pathways. Thus, sympathetic and embryonic DRG neurons possess parallel neurotrophic response mechanisms that may be triggered by different types of input stimuli.

Differences in Neurotrophic Activity of Various cAMP Derivatives

Our data indicate that 8-substituted cAMP derivates are much more effective than N^6-substituted analogs in sustaining neuronal survival. The two types of derivatives have different conformations; C8-substituted analogs have a predominantly "syn" configuration while N^6-substituted derivatives possess an "anti" configuration (Hoppe and Wagner, 1974; Hoppe et al., 1978). This, in turn, may result in the two types of derivatives having differential interaction with one or more specific binding sites for cAMP that are involved in a neurotrophic pathway. There is already in the literature evidence that a given cAMP-binding site may show different affinities for C8- and N^6-substituted analogs (Lohmann and Walter, 1984; Ogreid et al., 1985; Rannels and Corbin, 1980) and that the two types of derivatives may elicit different types of responses in the same cell type (Lohmann and Walter, 1984).

One may speculate that the capacity of a given neuron to respond to cAMP and its derivatives as neurotrophic agents requires that a particular cAMP-binding site or set of sites be present at appropriate abundance. This may explain why CPT-cAMP fails to elicit neurite outgrowth from the NGF-responsive PC12 line of rat pheochromocytoma cells (Greene and Shooter, 1980). It also appears in some cells that, for reasons which are not presently well understood, the N^6-substituted analogs may exert effective neurotrophic action. This seems to be the case for a subpopulation of sympathetic neurons as described here and for murine neuroblastoma cells (Prasad, 1975).

The observed differential neurotrophic activities of the C8- and N^6-substituted analogs raise an important caveat for experiments designed to assay the biological activities of cAMP derivatives. That is, it is important to test *both* classes of analogs for functional activity. Otherwise, one might incorrectly conclude that a given cellular response cannot be evoked by exposure to cAMP and its derivatives.

The Presence of Multiple Neurotrophic Response Mechanisms in a Single Type of Neuron

Our findings indicate that a single type of neuron may possess the capacity to respond to more than one type of neurotrophic input via the presence of parallel pathways. This may mean, as in the case of neurotransmission, that multiple neurotrophic inputs may be integrated. Such an occurrence could provide for additive and potentiative effects as well as permit a wide range of more subtle modulation of response. Thus, the extent of expression of a variety of neuronal phenotypic properties may reflect the cumulative input of multiple neurotrophic influences. This would significantly extend the degree of behavioral plasticity of a given neuron.

Possible Significance and Consequences of the Presence of a cAMP-Responsive Neurotrophic Pathway in NGF-Sensitive Neurons

There are several ways in which the present findings may be relevant to our understanding of the development of NGF-responsive neurons. For example, there are early developmental periods during which sympathetic and sensory neurons do not appear to require NGF for their survival or differentiation (Coughlin and Collins, 1985). It is conceivable that a cAMP-dependent mechanism may sustain these cells before they acquire a dependence upon NGF. Also, sympathetic neurons become less-and-less acutely dependent on NGF with increasing development (Gorin and Johnson, 1980), while maturing DRG neurons appear to lose their NGF requirement entirely. Again, it is possible that a cAMP-dependent neurotrophic mechanism is responsible for cell maintenance after the loss of the NGF requirement.

As noted above, it is also possible that the cAMP-responsive neurotrophic pathway normally functions in conjunction with other neurotrophic inputs, rather than as a singletary influence. Sympathetic neurons possess receptors for a number of agents that may raise their intracellular levels of cAMP. One can envision that the release of such agents during neurotransmission may lead to long-term neurotrophic actions.

Our findings also have several practical implications. One is for study of the NGF mechanism. Among the difficulties in working out the NGF mechanism with sympathetic neurons is that such cells require NGF for survival. Hence, it is not directly possible to compare NGF-treated with control, non-treated sympathetic neurons. However, the use of 8-derivatized cAMP analogs should now provide cultures of viable mammalian sympathetic neurons to which NGF can subsequently be added. This should permit the direct study of both acute and long-term effects of NGF. Also, comparison of both the similarities and differences in neurotrophic responses to NGF and to cAMP derivatives should shed light on the mechanistic pathways involved in the actions of both of these agents. For instance, the most likely primary action of cAMP derivatives is the activation of protein kinases. The ability of such derivatives to mimic some aspects of the NGF response suggests that this factor may also function via the phosphorylation of proteins. Our findings further suggest, however, that such NGF-promoted phosphorylations do not occur via a cAMP-mediated pathway.

A second practical implication raised by this study is that 8-derivatized cAMP analogs may exert trophic effects on neuronal types in addition to sympathetic and sensory neurons. It will be important to test whether these compounds will support additional populations of NGF-responsive neurons such as those found in the forebrain, as well as a variety of neuronal types that do not appear to respond to NGF.

A third practical implication of our observations is that 8-substituted cAMP derivatives may be active as neurotrophic agents in vivo. If this were to be the case, then these compounds have the potential to be used to promote the repair and regeneration of sympathetic and sensory (and possibly other) nerves. In preliminary experiments, we have found that newborn rats can tolerate the injection of CPT-cAMP to whole body concentrations similar to those we employed in vitro.

A final potential exploitation of the neurotrophic actions of the 8-substituted cAMP derivatives is to ameliorate diseases resulting from a failure in any step of normal neurotrophic pathways. That is, such compounds may be used, via activation of a parallel neurotrophic pathway, to support neurons that lose the source of, or cannot respond to, their normal neurotrophic factors. One potential example is human familial dysautonomia. In this genetic developmental disease, sympathetic, sensory and parasympathetic neurons die (Pearson et al., 1971). One possible cause of this is a defect in responsiveness to neurotrophic factors such as NGF. It is possible that this defect can be corrected by application of appropriate cAMP derivatives. Conceivably other defects in which neuronal degeneration occurs (eg. Parkinson's and Alzheimer's diseases) may be ameliorated by activation of a cAMP-responsive neurotrophic pathway.

ACKNOWLEDGMENTS

We thank Dr. B. Jastorff for generously providing samples of Rp-cAMPS. This work was supported by grants from the US National Institutes of Health (NS-16036) and the Dysautonomia Foundation. R.E.R. was supported in part by NIH predoctoral training grant GM-07827.

REFERENCES

Coughlin MD, Collins MB (1985) Nerve growth factor-independent development of embryonic mouse sympathetic neurons in dissociated cell culture. Devl Biol 110:392-401.

Gorin PD, Johnson EM Jr (1980) Effects of long-term nerve growth factor deprivation on the nervous system of the adult rat: An experimental autoimmune approach. Brain Res 198:27-42.

Greene LA, Shooter EM (1980) The nerve growth factor: Biochemistry, synthesis, and mechanism of action. Ann Rev Neurosci 3:353-402.

Greene LA, Tischler AS (1982) PC12 pheochromocytoma cultures in neurobiological research. Adv Cell Neurobiol 3:373-414.

Hoppe J, Rieke E, Wagner KG (1978) Mechanism of activation of protein kinase I from rabbit skeletal muscle. Eur J Biochem 83:411-417.

Hoppe J, Wagner KG (1974) Synthesis and properties of N^6, C^8 and C^2 spin-labelled derivatives of adenosine cyclic 3':5'-monophosphate. Eur J Biochem 48:519-525.

Lohmann SM, Walter U (1984) Regulation of the cellular and subcellular concentrations and distribution of cyclic nucleotide-dependent protein kinases. Adv Cyclic Nucleotide Res Protein Phos 18:63-117.

Ogreid D, Ekanger R, Siva RH, Miller JP, Sturm P, Corbin JD, Doskeland SO (1985) Activation of protein kinase isozymes by cyclic nucleotide analogs used singly or in combination. Eur J Biochem 150:219-227.

Pearson J, Budzilovich G, Finegold MJ (1971) Sensory, motor and autonomic dysfunction: the nervous system in familial dysautonomia. Neurology 21:486-493.

Prasad KN (1975) Differentiation of neuroblastoma cells in culture. Biol Rev 50:129-265.

Rannels SR, Corbin JD (1980) Two different intrachain cAMP binding sites of cAMP-dependent protein kinases. J Biol Chem 155:7085-7088.

Richter-Landsberg C, Jastorff B (1986) The role of cAMP in nerve growth factor-promoted neurite outgrowth in PC12 cells. J Cell Biol 102:821-829.

Rothermel JD, Jastorff B, Botelho LHP (1984) Inhibition of glucagon-induced glycogenolysis in isolated rat hepatocytes by the Rp diastereomer of adenosine 3',5'-phosphorothioate. J Biol Chem 259:8151-8155.

Rothermel JD, Stec WJ, Baraniak J, Jastorff B, Botelho LHP (1983) Inhibition of glycogenolysis in isolated rat hepatocytes by the Rp diastereomer of adenosine cyclic 3',5'-phosphorothioate. J Biol Chem 258:12125-12128.

Rydel RE, Greene LA (1987) Cyclic AMP analogs promote survival and neurite outgrowth in cultures of rat sympathetic and sensory neurons independently of nerve growth factor. Proc Natl Acad Sci USA, in press.

Thoenen H, Edgar D (1985) Neurotrophic factors. Science 119:238-242.

Neuronal Plasticity and Trophic Factors
G. Biggio, P.F. Spano, G. Toffano, S.H. Appel, G.L. Gessa (eds.)
Fidia Research Series, Symposia in Neuroscience VII
Liviana Press, Padova © 1988

CHARACTERIZATION AND PURIFICATION
OF A STRIATAL-DERIVED NEURONOTROPHIC FACTOR (SDNF)

Giovanna Ferrari, Carlo Soranzo, Lanfranco Callegaro, Roberto Dal Toso, Daniela Benvegnú, Gino Toffano and Alberta Leon

Fidia Research Laboratories,
via Ponte della Fabbrica 3/A, 35031 Abano Terme, Italy

INTRODUCTION

During development, neuronal survival and death are closely related to the size of their target fields. This has led to the hypothesis that nerve cells are dependent for their growth and maintenance on the availability of specific neuronotrophic factors (Thoenen and Edgar, 1985; Crutcher, 1986). The best evidence by far for a neuron-target trophic interaction derives from the discovery of Nerve Growth Factor (NGF) (Levi Montalcini, 1966). This protein has long been known to play a critical role in supporting the survival, neurite outgrowth and expression of characteristic traits of sensory and sympathetic neurons during development (Greene and Shooter, 1980; Thoenen and Barde, 1980; Levi Montalcini and Calissano, 1986). The recent observation that NGF is able to prevent death also of adult lesioned cholinergic neurons in the basal forebrain has led to the suggestion that neuronotrophic factors may play an important role not only during development, but also in the adult, in particular following brain injury (Hefti, 1986; Williams et al., 1986; Korshing, 1986).

Since the action of NGF appears at present to address several distinct populations

---

Abbreviations: BZT: benztropine mesylate, CNS: central nervous system, DA: dopamine, DABA: L-2,4-dia-mino-butyric acid, GABA: γ-amino-butyric acid, GFAP: glial fibrillary acidic protein, GIF: glyoxylic acid-induced fluorescence, HPLC: high pressure liquid chromatography, NGF: nerve growth factor, SDNF: stria-tum-derived neuronotrophic factor.

of neurons, it is reasonable to believe that additional trophic factors exist for other types of neurons (Varon, 1985). While numerous trophic activities have been detected to date, only limited success has been achieved in purifying these substances to homogeneity (Barde et al., 1982; Barbin et al., 1984b; Gospodarowicz et al., 1984; Gurney et al., 1986). In general, these trophic proteins are seen to exert their effects on peripheral neurons. Information on factors influencing survival of specific CNS neuronal types and/or development (e.g. expression of neurotransmitter-related properties) is, in contrast, quite limited. To extend our efforts in this latter direction, we have attempted to purify and biologically characterize neuronotrophic activity detected in bovine caudate. For this purpose, dissociated foetal mesencephalic cells were utilized as a bioassay system. Data available indicate that the neuronotrophic activity is associated with a fraction whose main component is a basic protein of $\approx$ 14,000 molecular weight (M.W.).

In the following we will briefly summarize: (a) the characteristics of the in vitro bioassay system; (b) the relative parameters utilized to monitor trophic activity present in crude and semi-purified extracts from bovine caudate; and (c) the procedures employed to purify and biologically characterize the trophic activity. Most of the techniques used in this study have been described elsewhere (Dal Toso et al., in press).

Characteristics of the Bioassay System Utilized

A valid strategy for the detection and characterization of neuronotrophic factors in the CNS requires the establishment of systems based on the utilization of primary dissociated CNS cell cultures (Barbin et al., 1984a). However, in view of the cellular heterogeneity in these cultures, such systems only allow for a gross evaluation of morphological and functional neuronal properties unless non-neuronal influences are limited, specific neuronal populations identified and cell-specific behaviors assessed. As already mentioned, dissociated foetal (E_{13}) mouse mesencephalic cell cultures were utilized to quantify the trophic activity present in the bovine caudate extracts. Culture conditions and parameters assessed were selected so as to satisfy the above criteria.

In particular, mesencephalic cells were maintained in a serum-free, hormone supplemented medium to avoid proliferation of nonneuronal cells, which may overwhelm the nondividing neurons and mask specific influences produced in or added to the culture (Di Porzio et al., 1980). At 4 days in culture, less than 2% of the cells were immunoreactive to glial fibrillary acidic protein (GFAP) antiserum. In contrast, 98% of the cells were labelled with RT97, a monoclonal antibody which recognizes the 145-200 Kd neurofilament protein subunits. Most of the stained cells had very long and branched processes.

Furthermore, due to the heterogeneity of the neuronal cells present in the cultures, attention was focused on the dopaminergic and gabaergic neurons. For example, the number of dopaminergic neurons was evaluated, following catecholamine uptake, utilizing the glyoxylic acid-induced fluorescence (GIF) technique (Bolstad et al., 1979). Approximately 0.15% of the attached mesencephalic cells after 4 days in culture could be visualized by this technique. These cells had fusiform or multipolar somata displaying long and branched neurites. The GIF+ neurons were still present after the addition of desmethylimipramine or fluoxetine but absent after benztropine mesylate (BZT), suggesting that most, if not all, of the GIF$^+$ neurons possess dopaminergic characteristics. In addition, we followed these neurons biochemically by assessing the BZT-sensitive ^{3}H-dopamine (DA) uptake as a function of time. To avoid a cell density-dependent masking of survival, we chose to work within a cell density range producing a linear increase of DA uptake. As illustrated in Figure 1, when 1×10^6 cells are seeded per 35 mm plate, the BZT-sensitive DA uptake reaches a maximum value at day 4 and then declines at day 8. The decline in the extent of DA uptake is closely related to a decline in the number of GIF positive neurons. This indicates that the uptake parameter is a good index to quantify not only cell development (maturation of characteristic neurotransmitter-linked traits), but also survival. Similar results were obtained measuring the L-2,4-diamino-butyric acid (DABA)-sensitive ^{14}C-γ-amino-butyric-acid (GABA) uptake, suggesting analogous behaviors of the different neuronal cell types present in the culture.

SDNF: Purification Procedure

Preliminary experiments utilizing adult rat striatum showed that a supernatant fraction (100,000 g × 60 min) contained activity capable of increasing, in a concentration-dependent manner, both specific ^{3}H-DA and ^{14}C-GABA uptake at day 4 (10^6

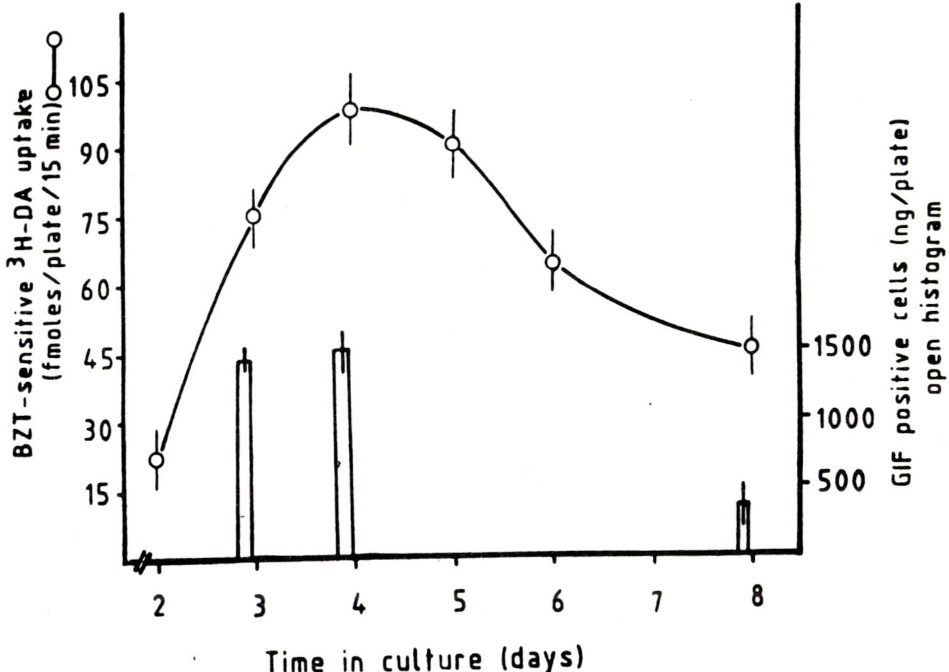

Figure 1. GIF$^+$ cells and BZT-sensitive DA uptake as a function of time in vitro. Mesencephalic cells were seeded at a density of 1×10^6 cells/35 mm dish. BZT-sensitive DA uptake (————); number GIF$^+$ cells (open histograms).

cells seeded/35 mm dish). This activity was resistant to acid treatment (pH 4.5, 2 hours) and was non-dialyzable (cut off 8×10^3). Since bovine caudate showed similar results (see below) and could be obtained in large quantities, this source was subsequently routinely utilized for identification and purification of the biologically active material.

The purification procedure employed is as reported by Dal Toso et al. (in press) and consists essentially of three major steps. In brief, an acid-precipitated and dialyzed crude supernatant fraction obtained from bovine caudate (step 1) was applied to a Sephadex G-150 column (step 2). Neuronotrophic activity was found to elute in the range of approximately $10\text{-}30 \times 10^3$ M.W. These active fractions were further purified by high pressure liquid chromatography (HPLC) using an ion exchange TSK-CM-3SW column (step 3). Figure 2 shows a typical HPLC elution profile. Trophic activity was found to occur only in association with the last protein peak, eluting with 1M ammonium acetate. This elution profile is similar to that generally seen with basic protein(s) (isoelectric point (IP) $\gtrsim$ 10). Silver staining of SDS gels of the active HPLC fraction showed the presence of only one band with a molecular weight of $\approx$ 14,000, henceforth called striatum derived neuronotrophic factor (SDNF). See Table 1 for protein recovery achieved following each of the major purification steps.

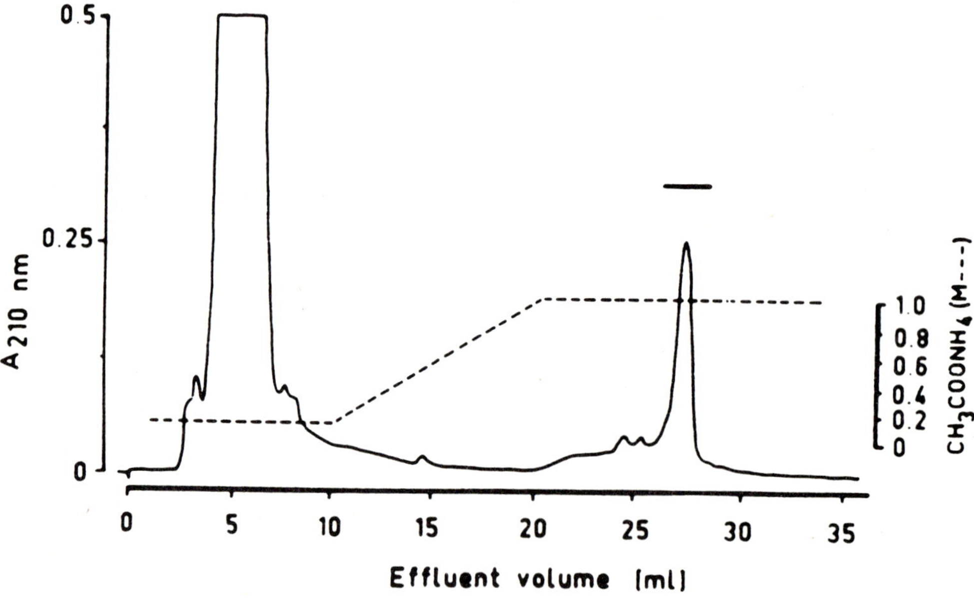

Figure 2. HPLC chromatography utilizing TSK-CM-3SW column of the active fractions obtained from the Sephadex G-150 column: elution profile monitored at 210 nm. The column was eluted sequentially with an ammonium acetate gradient utilizing 0.1 M - ammonium acetate (pH 6.5) (Buffer A) and 1 M ammonium acetate pH 6.5 (Buffer B) as follows: 100% A - 0% B (isocratic) 0% A - 100% B (linear), and 0% A - 100% B (isocratic). All fractions were assessed for their ability to increase specific neurotransmitter uptake in the mesencephalic cells. Activity was found in eluates depicted by the horizontal bar.

Table 1. *Purification and recovery of neuronotrophic activity from bovine caudate nuclei**

Purification step**	Protein recovery (mg)	Specific activity (µg prot/trophic unit)	Fold-purification
Supernatant	750	10.00	1
Sephadex G 150	3.5	0.30	33
TSK-CM-3SW	0.24	0.01	1000

*   starting material $\approx$ 150 g of caudate tissue

** see text for further elucidations

SDNF: Biological Activity

Adding to the cultures, at plating time, the acid-precipitated and dialyzed crude supernatant extract obtained from bovine caudate caused, when assayed at day 4, a concentration-dependent increase of BZT-sensitive DA uptake. Maximal increases were observed following addition of 40 µg protein/ml culture medium. The supernatant extract increased in a similar way also the DABA-sensitive GABA uptake, indicating that the effects on the various neuronal populations in the cultures were not cell specific. Analogous results were observed at day 8, and at that time the effects on the uptake parameters coincided with a significant reduction in the overall loss of the number of adhering cells. Total DNA content of treated cultures (40 µg protein/ml) was 2-3 times higher than that of control cultures treated with equivalent amounts of serum albumin. In addition, the number of GIF$^+$ neurons was three times higher in the presence of the striatal extract (Fig. 3).

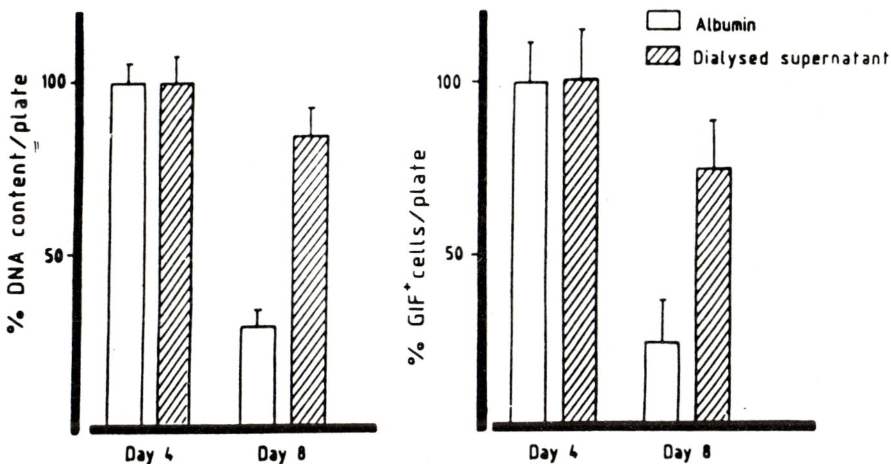

Figure 3. Effect of dialysed supernatant on DNA content and number of GIF$^+$ cells with time in culture. See text for further details.

Similar results regarding the uptake parameters and cell survival were also observed following addition of the active eluate(s) obtained following Sephadex G-150 (step 2) and HPLC cation-exchange chromatography (step 3). The only difference was in the amount of protein necessary for half-maximal stimulation of the uptake parameters. In particular, since the effects on the uptake parameters permitted a precise quantitative analysis and was correlated at all times with cell survival, we defined one trophic unit as that amount of protein (μg/ml) necessary to give half-maximal stimulation of the uptake parameters. Table 1 reports the specific trophic activity evaluated at each of the purification steps. The fold-purification achieved in terms of biological activity is about 1000-fold with respect to the starting supernatant (half maximal activities of 10 μg/ml and 10 ng/ml after step 1 and step 3, respectively).

CONCLUSION

The results reported show that extracts from bovine caudate contain activity capable of increasing high affinity neurotransmitter uptake parameters and cell survival of at least the dopaminergic and gabaergic neurons present in the mesencephalic culture system utilized. Purification procedures indicate that this trophic activity is associated with a fraction whose main component is a basic protein of approximately 14,000 M.W. This latter material, designated as striatum-derived neuronotrophic factor (SDNF), increases in a dose-dependent manner (half-maximal activity of $\approx$ 10 ng/ml) the development of both the cultured mesencephalic dopaminergic and gabaergic neurons. In addition, SDNF prevents normally occurring cell loss over time.

Noteworthy is that SDNF exerts a trophic effect not only on the dopaminergic but also on other neurons, e.g. gabaergic, present in the culture system. This neuronal aspecificity may be simply a reflection of the presence of more than one neuronotrophic agent in the preparation utilized or, alternatively, may be due to the cell heterogeneity and multiplicity of the neuronal development stages in the cultures. In addition, we cannot, at present, exclude the possibility that SDNF might act primarily on nonneuronal cells, in turn supporting neuronal survival. However, the low density of astrocytes in our cultures and the observed effects at early times argue against an indirect effect of this kind.

Furthermore, despite the chemical similarities to NGF, SDNF is clearly distinguishable from male mouse salivary gland ß-NGF. In particular:

— the addition of NGF at concentrations ranging from 1 to 300 ng/ml is totally ineffective in modifying the uptake parameters and cell survival of the mesencephalic cells;

— antibodies to NGF fail to abolish the SDNF effects on the above parameters; and

— SDNF is active in promoting neurite regeneration in NGF-primed cells replaced in the absence of NGF, an effect not blocked by antibody against NGF (Ferrari G., unpublished observations). However, since the discovery of NGF, other neuronotrophic factors directed towards CNS neurons have been isolated and characterized (Kligman, 1982; Müller et al., 1984; Kligman and Marshak, 1985; Turner, 1985a; 1985b; Johnson et al., 1986; Morrison et al., 1986; Tomozawa and Appel, 1986; Walicke et al., 1986; Mizrachi et al., 1986). Currently we are examining the possibility that SDNF may resemble or contain one or more identified growth factor activities.

ACKNOWLEDGMENTS

We are extremely grateful to Drs G. Kirschner and S.D. Skaper for active participation during the course of the work and the preparation of the manuscript. We also thank C. Minozzi for technical assistance and A. Bedeschi for typing the manuscript.

REFERENCES

Barbin G, Selak I, Manthorpe M, Varon S (1984a) Use of central neuronal cultures for the detection of neuronotrophic agents. Neuroscience 12:33-43.

Barbin G, Manthorpe M, Varon S (1984b) Purification of the chick eye ciliary neuronotrophic factor. J Neurochem 43:1468-1478.

Barde Y-A, Edgar D, Thoenen H (1982) Purification of a new neurotrophic factor from mammalian brain. EMBO J 1:549-553.

Bolstad G, Kalland T, Srebro B, Stene-Larsen G (1979) Modifications of the glyoxylic acid method for visualization of catecholamines in vertebrate and invertebrate species. Comp Biochem Physiol 62:61-65.

Crutcher KA (1986) The role of growth factors in neuronal development and plasticity. Crit Rev Clin Neurobiol 2:297-333.

Dal Toso R, Giorgi O, Soranzo C, Kirschner G, Ferrari G, Favaron M, Benvegnú D, Presti D, Vicini S, Toffano G, Azzone GF, Leon A (1987) Development and survival of neurons in dissociated fetal mesencephalic serum-free cell cultures: I. Effects of cell density of an adult mammalian striatal derived neuronotrophic factor (SDNF). J Neurosci, in press.

Di Porzio U, Daguet MC, Glowinski J, Prochiantz A (1980) Effect of striatal cells on in vitro maturation of mesencephalic dopaminergic neurons grown in serum-free conditions. Nature 288: 370-373.

Gospodarowicz D, Cheng J, Lui G-M, Baird A, Bohlen P (1984) Isolation by heparin sepharase affinity chromatography of brain fibroblast growth factor: identity with pituitary fibroblast growth factor. Proc Natl Acad Sci USA 81: 6963-6967.

Greene LA, Shooter EM (1980) The nerve growth factor: biochemistry synthesis and mechanism of action. Annu Rev Neurosci 3: 353-402.

Gurney ME, Heinrich SP, Lee MR, Yin H-S (1986) Molecular cloning and expression of neuroleukin, a neuronotrophic factor for spinal and sensory neurons. Science 234: 566-574.

Hefti F (1986) Nerve growth factor promotes survival of septal cholinergic neurons after fimbrial transection. J Neurosci 6: 2155-2162.

Johnson JE, Barde YA, Schwab M, Thoenen H (1986) Brain-derived neuronotrophic factor supports the survival of cultured rat retinal ganglion cells. J Neurosci 6: 3031-3038.

Kligman D (1982) Isolation of a protein from bovine brain which promotes neurite extension from chick embryo cerebral cortex neurons in defined medium. Brain Res 250: 93-100.

Kligman D, Marshak DR (1985) Purification and characterization of a neurite extension factor from bovine brain. Proc Natl Acad Sci USA 82: 7136-7139.

Korsching S (1986) The role of nerve growth factor in the CNS. TINS 9: 570-573.

Levi Montalcini R (1966) The nerve growth factor: its mode of action on sensory and sympathetic nerve cells. Harvey Lect 60: 217-259.

Levi-Montalcini R, Calissano P (1986) Nerve growth factors as a paradigm for other polypeptide growth factors. TINS 9: 473-477.

Mizrachi Y, Rubinstein M, Kimbi Y, Schwartz M (1986) A neuronotrophic factor from goldfish brain: characterization and purification. J Neurochem 46: 1675-1682.

Morrison RS, Sharma A, de Vellis J, Bradshaw RA (1986) Basic fibroblast growth factor supports the survival of cerebral cortical neurons in primary culture. Proc Natl Acad Sci USA 83: 7537-7541.

Müller HW, Beckh S, Seifert W (1984) Neurotrophic factor for central neurons. Proc Natl Acad Sci USA 81: 1248-1252.

Thoenen H, Barde Y-A (1980) Physiology of nerve growth factor. Physiol Rev 60: 1284-1335.

Thoenen H, Edgar D (1985) Neuronotrophic factors. Science 225: 238-242.

Tomozawa Y, Appel SH (1986) Soluble striatal extracts enhance development of mesencephalic dopaminergic neurons in vitro. Brain Res 339: 111-124.

Turner JE (1985a) Neurotrophic stimulation of fetal rat retinal explant neurite outgrowth and cell survival: age-dependent relationships. Dev Brain Res 18: 251-263.

Turner JE (1985b) Promotion of neurite outgrowth and cell survival in dissociated fetal rat retinal cultures by a fraction derived from a brain extract. Dev Brain Res 18: 265-274.

Varon S (1985) Factors promoting the growth of the neurons system. In: Discussions in Neurosciences. Vol 2, n° 3, pp. 1-62.

Walicke P, Cowan WM, Ueno N, Baird A, Guillemin R (1986) Fibroblast growth factor promotes survival of dissociated hippocampal neurons and enhances neurite extension. Proc Natl Acad Sci USA 83: 3012-3016.

Williams LR, Varon S, Peterson GM, Victorin K, Fischer W, Björklund A, Gage FH (1986) Continuous infusion of nerve growth factor prevents basal forebrain neuronal death after fimbria-fornix transection. Proc Natl Acad Sci USA 83: 9231-9235.

Neuronal Plasticity and Trophic Factors
G. Biggio, P.F. Spano, G. Toffano, S.H. Appel, G.L. Gessa (eds.)
Fidia Research Series, Symposia in Neuroscience VII
Liviana Press, Padova © 1988

A SERUM FACTOR INDUCING NEURITE OUTGROWTH AND CELL ADHESION IN CEREBELLAR GRANULE CELLS

D. Mercanti, M.T. Ciotti and P. Calissano

Institute of Neurobiology, CNR, via Romagnosi 18a, 00196 Roma, Italy

INTRODUCTION

The discovery of Nerve Growth Factor (NGF) (Levi Montalcini and Hamburger, 1951; Levi Montalcini et al., 1954) brought to light the existence of a whole family of polypeptide growth factors having distinct types of target cells (Calissano et al., 1984; Levi Montalcini and Calissano, 1986). NGF remains, however, up to now, the only protein whose trophic and differentiative role for certain cells of the peripheral and central nervous system has been unequivocally established with in vivo experiments. Thus, while the action of a variety of polypeptides on in vitro explanted nerve cells has been reported (Thoenen and Edgar, 1985), nothing is known about their actual role in the intact animal.

We have adopted a strategy for the search of putative NGF-like factors based on two major criteria:

1. Highly stringent culture conditions allowing survival and possible differentiation of target cells *only* in the presence of the putative factor. To this aim, we have employed Eagle Basal Medium devoid of serum or of any of the substances (insulin, transferrin, putrescine) devised by Bottenstein and Sato to supplement a chemically defined medium (CDM) (Bottenstein and Sato, 1979).

2. Choice of an abundant, homogeneous population of nerve cells exhibiting a fast

---

Abbreviations: NOAF: neurite outgrowth adhesion factor, GFAP: glial fibrillary acidic protein, CDM: chemically defined medium, BME: basal medium (eagle), PGF: polypeptide growth factor, CNS: central nervous system.

response to the putative polypeptide growth factor(s). Granule cells dissociated from 8-day-old rat cerebella and cultured in vitro were the cells of choice for their correspondence to these requirements.

We report in this paper the identification and partial purification of a proteic factor that promotes neurite outgrowth and fasciculation as well as adhesion of cerebellar granule cells. These findings prospect the possibility of isolating for the first time a PGF acting on cerebellar granule cells as well as on other CNS neurons.

MATERIAL AND METHODS

Cerebellar granule cells dissociated from eight-day postnatal Wistar rats were cultured on poly-l-lysine coated, 12 mm diameter, round glass coverslips (four coverslips in each 35 mm Petri dish) for immunofluorescence studies.

Biological assays on fractions derived from purification steps were run on cells plated on 24 or 48 wells tissue culture dishes (Costar). Cerebella were dissociated and granule cells collected and seeded in serum-free Eagle Basal Medium (Gibco). Cells were plated at a density of 3×10^5 cell per square centimeter in BME (Gibco) and incubated at 37°C with 5% CO_2 in a humidified incubator.

Rabbit sera were collected from plasma clots, heat inactivated at 56°C for 30 minutes and stored at -20°C until use. Under these conditions full activity is retained for at least six months. Serum and the partially purified active fractions can be sterile-filtered through 0.22 filters (Millipore GS). Indirect immunofluorescence studies were performed as previously described (Levi et al., 1984; Gallo et al., 1986). Anti-GFAP was a gift of A. Bignami; anti-Synapsin I was a gift of P. De Camillis and anti-A_2B_5 was a gift of S. Alemà; anti-N-CAM like (F3) protein was a generous gift of Dr. Ceccarini.

RESULTS

Identification of Rabbit Serum as the Richest Source of a Factor Active on Cerebellar Granule Cells

During the course of an investigation on a placenta derived growth factor acting on cerebellar astrocytes (Mercanti et al., 1987), we found that rabbit sera had a very strong activity in promoting cerebellar granule cells association and neurite outgrowth and fasciculation (Fig. 1). A subsequent screening with varying concentrations of six distinct sera, derived from different species (fetal calf, horse, goat, rat, chick and human serum), confirmed the finding that rabbit serum has an activity 20-50 times higher than all other samples tested, with the exception of the human serum that exhibits a somewhat similar action. Such activity is characterized by two major properties (see Figs. 1 and 2):

— induction of granule cells association to form clusters or clumps composed of several cells;

— induction of a rapid and massive neurite outgrowth and fasciculation; the higher

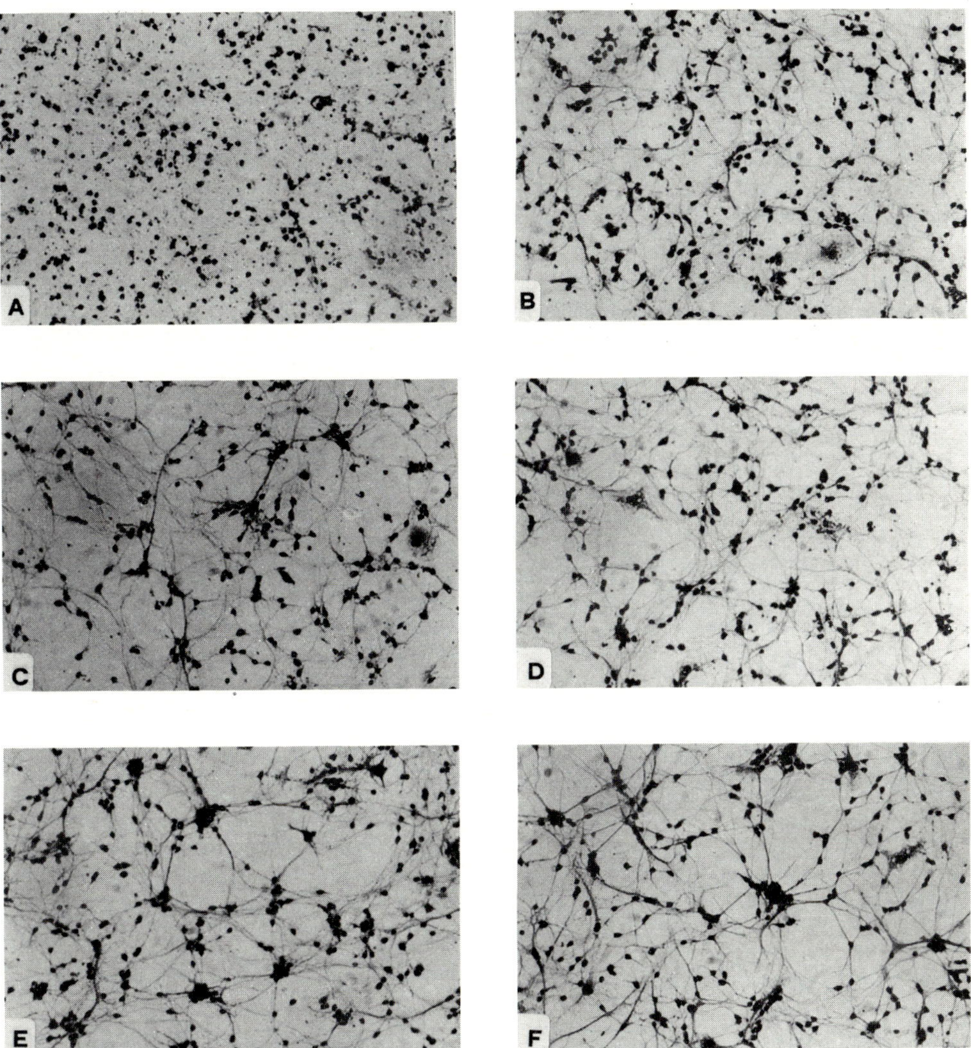

Figure 1. Effect of increasing concentration of rabbit serum on 8-day-old rat cerebellar granule cells in cultures. Cells were prepared as described in methods and cultured in BME containing 2 μl (B), 5 μl (C), 10 μl (D), 20 μl (E), 40 μl (F) of rabbit sera per milliliter of incubation media. Panel A represents control cultures without serum. After three days of incubation, cultures were fixed and stained as described (Gallo et al., 1986).

the concentration of rabbit or human sera, the larger and thicker the fascicles that several associated neurites form already after 1-2 days of incubation (Figs. 1 and 2).

In view of these effects, the substance(s) responsible for these activities has been operationally defined as neurite outgrowth adhesion factor (NOAF). Rabbit sera were thus chosen as the richest source of NOAF to be purified and characterized.

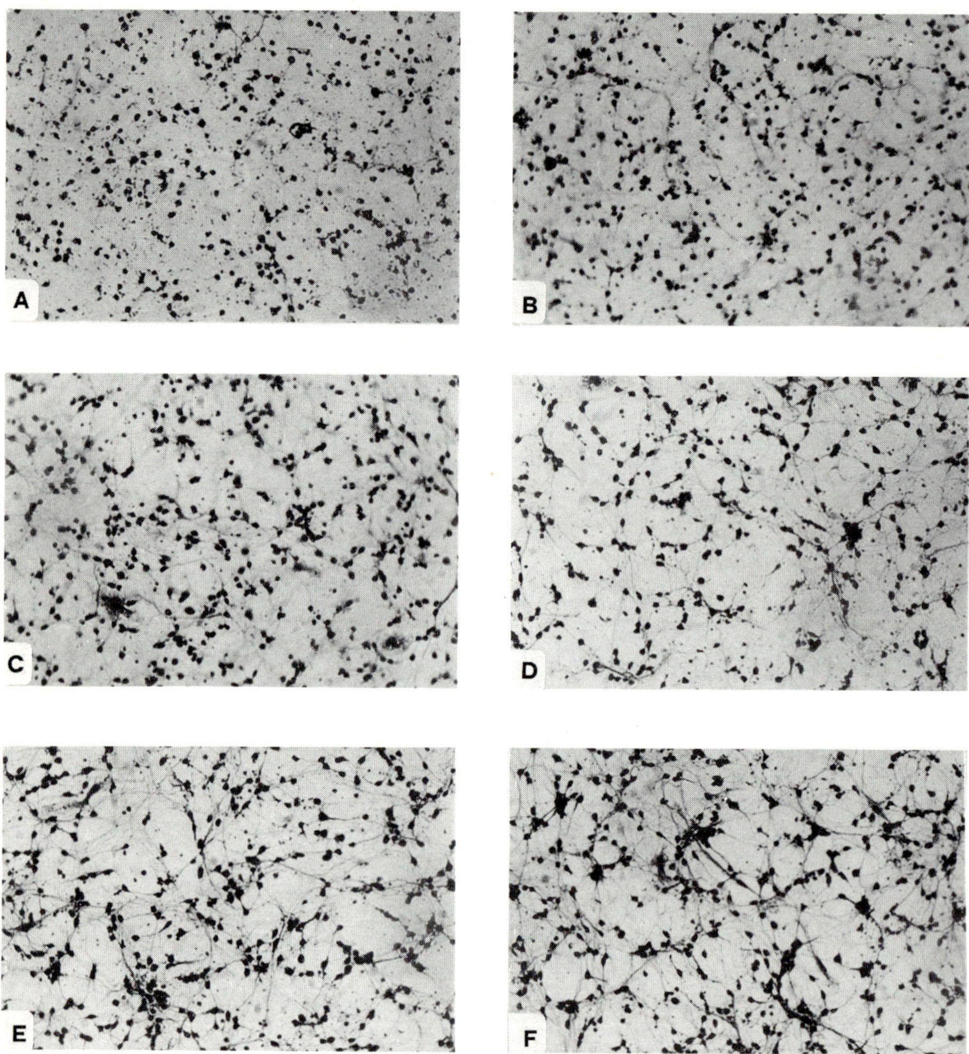

Figure 2. Effect of increasing concentrations of human serum on 8-day-old rat dissociated cerebellar granule cells. Cultures conditions, incubation time and serum concentrations are identical to those reported in Figure 1.

Preparation and Partial Characterization of NOAF

Several chromatographic procedures have been attempted to devise a purification protocol allowing at least a partial isolation of NOAF. These included ion exchange chromatography, gel filtration on Sephadex G-200, affinity chromatography on specific ligands such as protein A, heparin sulfate, gelatin as well as high pressure liquid chromatography both on cationic and anionic matrices. We are presently able to obtain a preparation that is 4-8000 fold purified over fetal calf sera and 2-400 fold purified compared to the specific activity of the whole rabbit sera. This preparation is obtained after five steps of fractionation involving gel-filtration over Sephadex G-200, followed by chromatography on gelatin-sepharose, protein-A-sepharose and heparin sulfate-sepharose. The NOAF activity flows through protein-A and gelatin sepharose columns and is retained by the heparin moiety from which is eluted at a .15 M NaCl concentration. The heparin eluate is finally electrophoresed under non-denaturing conditions with 10% acrylamide gel at pH 8.3 and the active fraction, mainly confined to the first 2 mm of the top of the gel, is eluted from the acrylamide matrix and can be directly used for tissue cultures or tests on its chemical nature. Table 1 summarizes some of the chemico-physical properties of NOAF.

Table 1. *Properties of partially purified NOAF*

M.W. (native) 50-100 kD	Not inhibited by anti-EGF
Heat labile (80 C, 10 min.)	Not inhibited by anti-PDGF
Digested with trypsin	Not inhibited by anti-NGF
Weak binding heparin-seph.	Not inhibited by anti-N-CAM
No binding to prot. A-seph.	Not inhibited by anti-Ng-CAM
No binding to gelatin-seph.	Not inhibited by anti-CAM-like

As can be seen, NOAF has an apparent molecular weight of 50-100 kD under non-denaturing conditions, is heat labile and its activity is destroyed by incubation with trypsin, pointing to its proteic nature. The binding to heparin suggests, but does not prove, that NOAF is a glycoprotein while the finding that it does not bind to protein-A or gelatin indicates that it does not belong to the vast majority of immunoglobulins nor to fibronectin. Furthermore, NOAF activity is not inhibited by antibodies directed against Epidermal Growth Factor (EGF), Platelet Derived Growth Factor (PDGF), Nerve Growth Factor (NGF) nor by antibodies directed against cell adhesion molecules (CAM) expressed both on nerve and glial cells.

Properties of the Rat Cerebellar Granule Cells Grown with NOAF

A major drawback of cultures of granule cells grown in 10% fetal calf sera or in a chemically defined medium is the proliferation of a vast number of glial cells, especially during a prolonged period of incubations, even when an antimitotic such as Ara-C is present in the culture medium.

When cerebellar granule cells are grown in 0.5% rabbit serum, or, even more impressively, with the partially purified NOAF, the number of GFAP cells is comparable to that of control cultures (Fig. 3, A-B). Although we do not have, up to now, a precise quantitative estimate of the actual reduction of glial cells under such

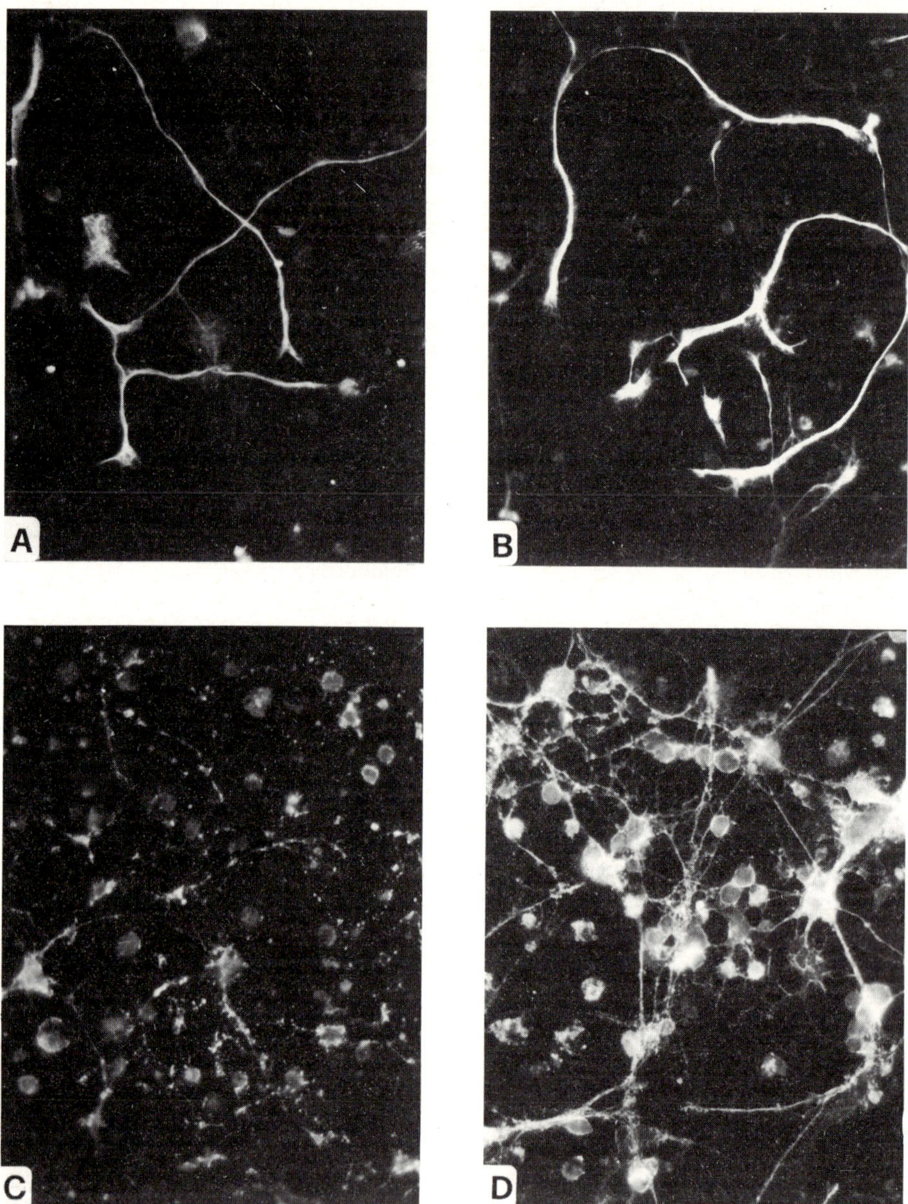

Figure 3. Indirect immunofluorescence staining performed with antibodies directed against GFAP and A2B5 antigens. Dissociated granule cells from 8-day-old rats were grown for four days in the absence (A-C) or in the presence (B-D) of a partially purified preparation of NOAF. Cultures (A-B) were fixed, permeabilized, treated with rabbit anti GFAP and stained with rhodamine conjugated goat anti rabbit antibodies. Sister cultures (C-D) were incubated with A2B5 monoclonal antibodies (ascite) and stained with fluorescein conjugated goat anti mouse antibodies followed by fixation.

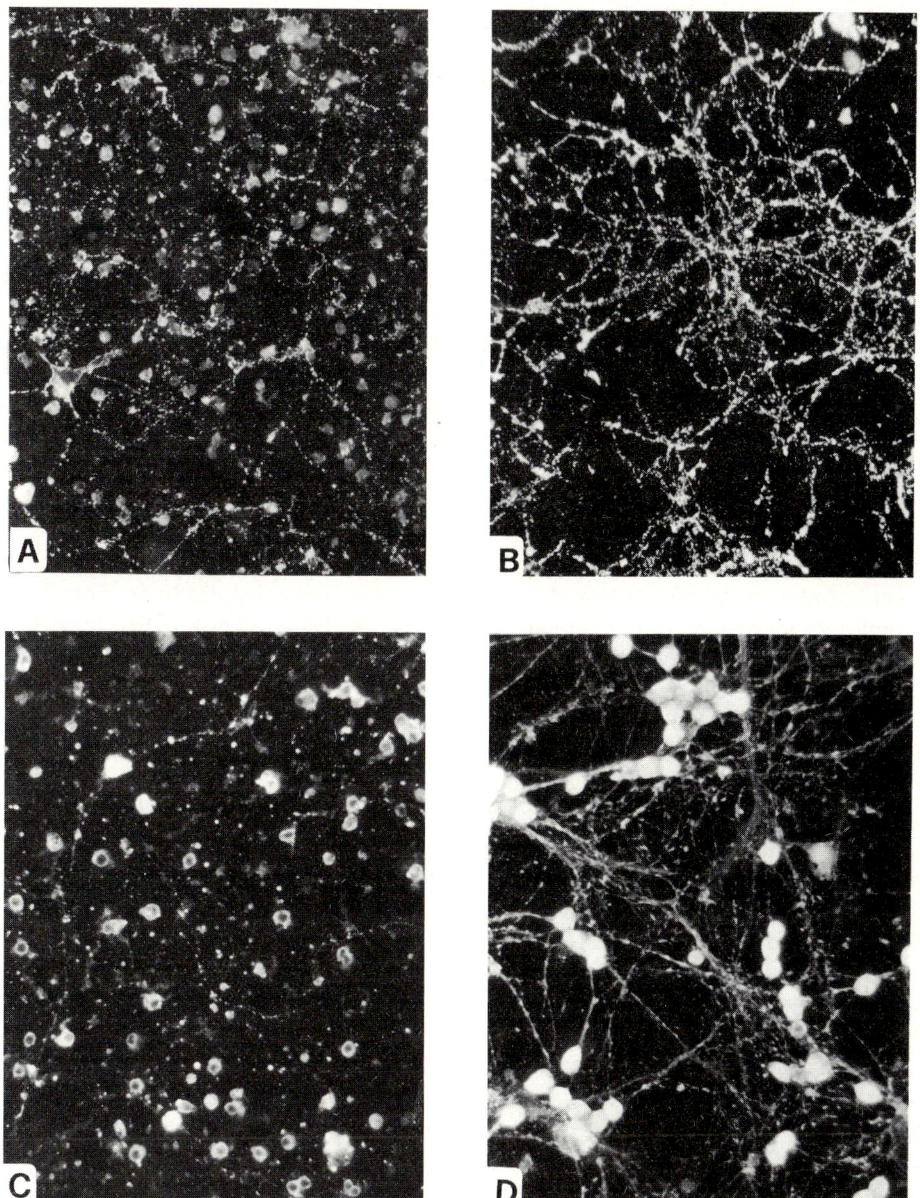

Figure 4. Indirect immunofluorescence staining performed with antibodies directed against tetanus toxin and synapsin I. Dissociated granule cells from eight-day-old rats were grown in the absence (A-C) or in the presence (B-D) of a partially purified preparation of NOAF for four days. Cells were treated with tetanus toxin (A-B) followed by incubation with horse anti tetanus toxin and fluoresceinated sheep anti horse antibodies. Sister cultures were fixed, permeabilized, incubated with rabbit anti synapsin I and stained with rhodamine conjugated goat anti rabbit antibodies (C-D).

conditions, indirect immunofluorescence studies strongly favor this conclusion (not shown).

Rat cerebellar granule cells grown with NOAF exhibit the usual morphology and express typical markers such as the antigen recognized by the monoclonal antibody A2B5 (Fig. 3, C-D).

Tetanus toxin binding on the perikaryon and on nerve processes is abundant and ubiquitous as in cells grown in a medium containing 10% fetal calf serum (not shown). The same is true also for synapsin I which is evenly expressed in granule cells cultured with NOAF (Fig. 4).

DISCUSSION

Some decades have elapsed since the elegant and unequivocal demonstration that survival and differentiation of some types of nerve cells are strictly dependent upon the continuous supply of a specific molecular entity which has become known as nerve growth factor, or NGF. This finding has prompted the search for other polypeptide growth factors (PGFs) acting on other neuronal and non-neuronal cells. Only non-neuronal PGFs, however, are presently specific, highly characterized factors, while the field of neuronotrophic factors has witnessed several abortive findings. Thus, while cell biologists have now in their hands factors such as EGF, PDGF, TGF, GM-CSF, whose sequences are well known and whose corresponding genes have been identified, neurobiologists can only exhibit NGF as their leader and paradigm, but have failed to identify and isolate PGFs whose physiological role has been unequivocally established.

This, of course, is not to be attributed to lack of competence or expertise. In our opinion, it is rather due to the much more difficult in vitro handling of nerve cells to be used as tests to set up ad hoc devised in vitro assays to quantitatively measure the presence and activity of a neuronotrophic factor. For example, while a mitogenic action can be precisely and easily assessed by thymidine incorporation or cell counting, neurite outgrowth, which is the most typical response of a differentiating neuron, is a relatively slow process which can be scored only in a semiquantitative fashion. It was thus mandatory to devise in vitro culture conditions that would give clear-cut and fast responses for the putative factor. We found that rat cerebellar granule cells cultures employed for the present studies perfectly fulfill these criteria. We were thus able to make rapid and quantitative screenings of potentially rich sources of a factor that is present in all sera tested but that is particularly abundant in rabbit serum. While the structural properties of NOAF are still unknown, further purification steps are necessary for its isolation in a pure form, its action on granule cells association, neurite outgrowth and fasciculation is fully evident. It remains to be established, possibly by the use of time-lapse cinematography, whether cell association occurs earlier and causes neurite outgrowth and fasciculation or, alternatively, whether they are independent processes. With highly purified preparations, it will be eventually possible to assess whether NOAF also plays some role in granule cell differentiation and migration in vivo. Only these experiments may ascertain whether NOAF is part of the large and ever-growing family of factors in search of an in vivo role or whether it belongs to the category of the few PGFs playing a physiological role in the differentiation and function of CNS neurons.

ACKNOWLEDGMENTS

This work has been supported by Progetto Finalizzato Oncologia and by Progetto Finalizzato Tecnologie Biomediche of Consiglio Nazionale delle Ricerche to P.C. We wish to thank Dr. R. Levi Montalcini for stimulating discussion during the preparation of the manuscript.

REFERENCES

Bottenstein JE, Sato GM (1979) Growth of a rat neuroblastoma cell line in serum-free supplemented medium. Proc Natl Acad Sci USA 76: 514.

Bignami A, Eng LF, Dahl D, Uyeda CT (1972) Localization of the glial fibrillary acidic protein in astrocytes by immunofluorescence. Brain Res 43: 429.

Calissano P, Cattaneo A, Aloe L, Levi Montalcini R (1984) The Nerve Growth Factor (NGF). Hormonal proteins and peptides Li CH, 12: 1-56.

Gallo V, Ciotti MT, Aloisi F, Levi G (1986) Developmental features of rat cerebellar neural cells cultured in a chemically defined medium. J Neurosci Res 15: 289.

Levi G, Aloisi F, Ciotti MT, Gallo V (1984) Autoradiographic Localization and Depolarization-Induced Release of Acidic Amino Acids in Differentiating Cerebellar Granule Cell Cultures. Brain Res 290: 77.

Levi Montalcini R, Calissano P (1986) Nerve Growth Factor as a paradigm for other polypeptide growth factors. Trends in Neurosciences (Oct): 473-477.

Levi Montalcini R, Hamburger V (1954) Selective growth stimulating effects of mouse sarcoma on sensory and sympathetic nervous system of the chick embryo. J Exp Zool 116: 321-362.

Levi Montalcini R, Meyer H, Hamburger V (1954) In vitro experiments on the effects of mouse sarcoma 180 and 37 on the spinal and sympathetic ganglia of the chick embryo. Cancer Res 14: 49-57.

Mercanti D, Luzzatto E, Ciotti MT, Levi G (1987) Mitogenic Effect of a Human Placental Factor on Astrocytes and Glial Precursors. Exp Cell Res 168: 182-190.

Raff MC, Fields KL, Hakomori S, Mirsky R, Pruss M, Winter J (1979) Cell type specific markers for distinguishing and studying neurons and the major classes of glial cells in culture. Brain Res 174: 283-308.

Thoenen H, Edgar D (1985) Neurotrophic Factors. Science 229: 238-248.

Neuronal Plasticity and Trophic Factors
G. Biggio, P.F. Spano, G. Toffano, S.H. Appel, G.L. Gessa (eds.)
Fidia Research Series, Symposia in Neuroscience VII
Liviana Press, Padova © 1988

APPLICATION OF GANGLIOSIDES, NERVE GROWTH FACTOR AND BRAIN TRANSPLANTS TO PREVENT CHOLINERGIC DEGENERATION IN THE CENTRAL NERVOUS SYSTEM

A. Claudio Cuello, Erik P. Pioro, Dusica Maysinger, Lorella Garofalo and Philip C. Tagari

Department of Pharmacology and Therapeutics,
McGill University, Montreal, Quebec, Canada, H3G 1Y6

INTRODUCTION

The mammalian neocortex receives a widespread distribution of cholinergic fibres, the majority of which seems to originate from the nucleus basalis magnocellularis (NBM) (Johnston et al., 1981; Fibiger, 1982; Cuello and Sofroniew, 1984). Immunohistochemical studies have demonstrated that this projection is apparently topographically organized in the cortex (Mesulam et al., 1986; Ingham et al., 1985). These fibres represent approximately 70% of the total cholinergic component of the cortex, the remainder deriving from local circuit neurons (Lehman et al., 1982; Johnston et al., 1981). Furthermore, neurons from the medial septal nucleus and nucleus of the vertical limb (diagonal band of Broca) provide an important cholinergic input to the hippocampus via the fimbria-fornix (Lewis and Shute, 1967; Oderfeld-Nowak et al., 1974; Meibach and Siegel, 1977).

Following the pivotal work of Rita Levi-Montalcini (Levi-Montalcini and

---

Abbreviations: CNS: central nervous system, NBM: nucleus basalis magnocellularis, C: cortex, S: septum, H: hippocampus, ChAT: choline acetyltransferase, GM_1: monosialoganglioside, NGF: nerve growth factor, NGFr: nerve growth factor receptor, i.p.: intraperitoneally, i.c.v.: intracerebroventricularly, mg: milligram, kg: kilogram.

Angeletti, 1968), it has been recently demonstrated that nerve growth factor (NGF) exerts trophic actions on specific cholinergic neurons in the rat central nervous system (CNS) (for review see Korsching, 1986). In particular, this has been illustrated in cholinergic basal forebrain neurons, both in vitro (Hefti et al., 1985; Honegger and Lenior, 1983) and in vivo (Gnahn et al., 1983; Hefti et al., 1984; Mobley et al., 1986). This is supported by evidence of NGF binding to receptors associated with these cholinergic neurons (Richardson et al., 1986; Raivich and Kreutzberg, 1987) and the identification of such NGF receptors (NGFr) using a monoclonal antibody (Taniuchi et al., 1986). In addition, the cortex is known to be a site of high NGF production possessing high levels of NGF messenger RNA (Korsching et al., 1985). Retrograde transport of NGF from neocortex to NBM (Seiler and Schwab, 1984) and from hippocampus to septum (Schwab et al., 1979) has been demonstrated in the rat. Dopaminergic neurons of the nigrostriatal pathway, in contrast, do not retrogradely transport NGF and are unresponsive to it (Schwab et al., 1979).

These findings in experimental animals shed new light on cortical-subcortical cholinergic interactions and support the suggestion that trophic factors may be involved in human neurodegenerative disorders such as Alzheimer's disease (Appel, 1981; Hefti, 1983). Cholinergic forebrain neurons are, in fact, markedly affected in this condition (Davies and Maloney, 1976; Perry et al., 1978; Rossor et al., 1982; Whitehouse et al., 1982; Bowen et al., 1983; Sims et al., 1983). In view of the above, it is conceivable that the cholinergic involvement in Alzheimer's disease represents a secondary effect from the loss of target sites and thereby depletion of relevant neurotrophic factors. Consistent with this proposal, we have obtained experimental evidence in the rat that forebrain cholinergic neurons are affected morphologically (Sofroniew et al., 1983b) and biochemically (Stephens et al., 1985) by cortical devascularizing lesions which deprive them of their major projection sites. We have been interested in preventing these secondary retrograde subcortical changes by applying various pharmacological therapies, including monosialoganglioside (GM_1) and NGF. More recently, however, we have used embryonic cortical cells implanted into the devascularized neocortex to replace the terminal projection field of cholinergic NBM neurons and thereby prevent their degeneration. Neural transplantation techniques have recently become important means of examining plasticity and regeneration in the lesioned mammalian CNS (for reviews, see Oblinger and Das, 1983; Kromer, 1983). Reversal of neurochemical and behavioural deficits in certain neurotransmitter systems has been achieved through implantation of embryonic donor neural tissue into specific lesioned regions of mammalian brain. This has been well shown in animal models of Parkinson's disease where functional effects of dopaminergic nigrostriatal pathway lesions have been reversed with embryonic substantia nigra implants (Dunnett et al., 1981).

ROLE OF GANGLIOSIDES AND NERVE GROWTH FACTOR
IN PROTECTING FOREBRAIN CHOLINERGIC NEURONS

Devascularization of the rat neocortex results in necrosis of the cortical area with preservation of subcortical structures. The retrograde degeneration of the NBM which results is reflected in specific morphological (Fig. 1b and c) and biochemical alterations

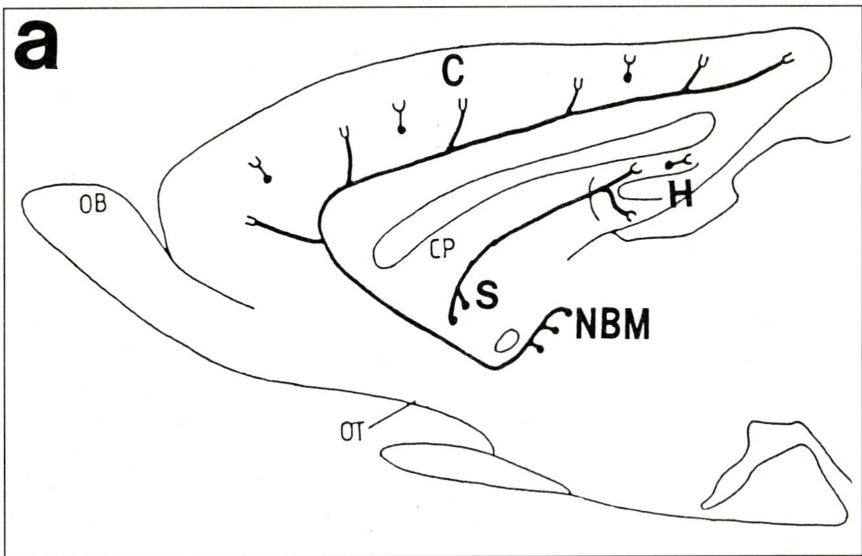

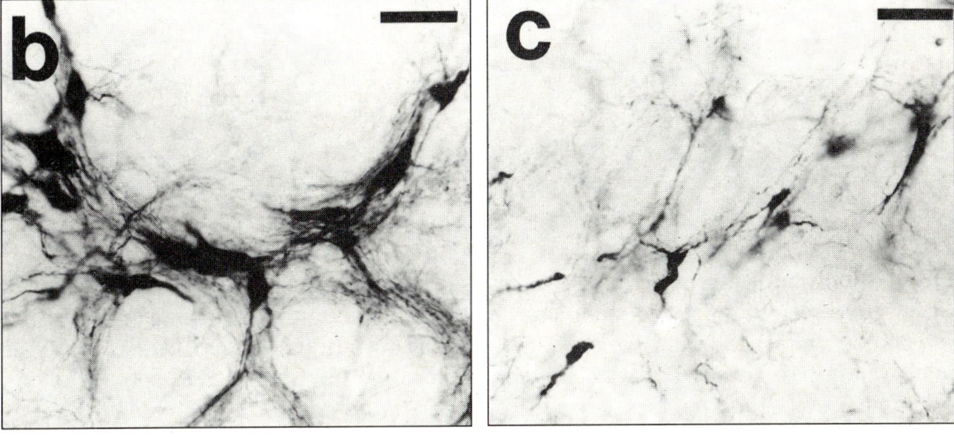

Figure 1. Morphological consequences of terminal field lesions on projecting basal forebrain cholinergic neurons. a) The projection of cholinergic neurons of the nucleus basalis magnocellularis (NBM) to cortex (C) and of the septum (S) to hippocampus (H) of the rat is represented diagrammatically (sagittal section). CP, caudate-putamen; OB, olfactory bulb; OT, olfactory tubercle. Animals were perfused with 4% paraformaldehyde and 50 micrometre free-floating sections were immunostained with monoclonal antibodies directed against ChAT (Eckenstein and Thoenen, 1982) and horseradish peroxidase (Cuello et al., 1984). b) ChAT immunopositive neurons in the NBM of a control animal. Scale bar = 100 micrometres. c) Retrograde degenerative changes in ipsilateral NBM cholinergic neurons 30 days after a unilateral cortical lesion resulted in a shrunken appearance and loss of cell processes. Scale bar = 100 micrometres. d) ChAT immunoreactive septal neurons from an unlesioned animal (coronal section). Scale bar = 1 millimeter. e) Ipsilateral degeneration with loss of immunostained cholinergic septal neurons was apparent 10 weeks after a suction lesion of the left hippocampus. Scale bar = 1 millimeter.

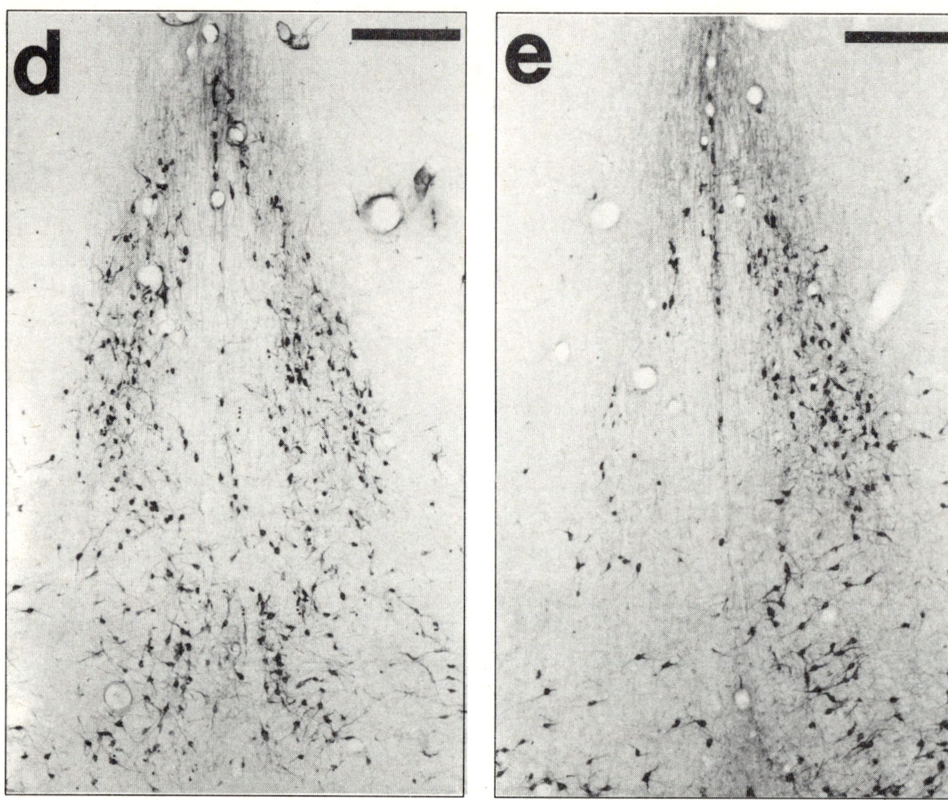

Figure 1. (Continued)

of its cortically-projecting cholinergic neurons. These changes are expressed as a reduction of cross-sectional area of cholinergic somata, a diminution of neuronal processes (Sofroniew et al., 1983b) and a depletion of choline acetyltransferase (ChAT) activity in the NBM but in no other CNS areas (Stephens et al., 1985). Similarly, retrograde involution and loss of septal nucleus cholinergic neurons results from the removal of the hippocampus (Fig. 1d and e).

The monosialoganglioside GM_1 has been reported to exert certain neurotrophic effects in vitro and in vivo (Gorio et al., 1983; Karpiak, 1983). In view of this, we have investigated the effects of GM_1 in the rat model of retrograde degeneration of forebrain neurons mentioned above. In our initial studies the daily intraperitoneal (i.p.) administration of 30 mg/kg of GM_1 to young rats with cortical lesions completely prevented the ipsilateral decrease in ChAT activity otherwise seen. When compared to vehicle injected controls, treatment with GM_1 caused an increase in ChAT enzymatic activity in both sham operated and cortically damaged animals (Table 1; from Cuello et al., 1986). The effects of chronic ganglioside administration on ChAT immunoreactive neurons of the medial septal nucleus and vertical limb of the diagonal band following unilateral hippocampal removal (Sofroniew et al., 1986a) were similarly examined. In this system, ganglioside administration arrested the cell losses observed in the ipsilateral

Table 1. *The effect of chronic ganglioside GM_1 treatment on ChAT activity in microdissected NBM from animals with unilateral (right) cortical lesions*

	Left			Right		
	ChAT	S.E.M.	n	ChAT	S.E.M.	n
Sham operated vehicle inj.	52.7	5.3	5	49.4	4.3	5
Sham operated GM_1	97.4**	6.6	6	83.1**	5.7	6
Operated vehicle inj.	54.5	5.4	5	43.0*	2.5	5
Operated GM_1	70.7**	3.7	6	75.4**	5.0	6

Choline acetyltransferase activity (nmols ACh/mg protein/hour) was measured in the ipsilateral (right) and contralateral (left) nucleus basalis from cortically lesioned or sham operated young animals after treatment for 30 days with GM_1 or vehicle (saline).
*, $p < 0.01$; **, $p < 0.001$.

side of these structures. Table 1 summarizes these findings in the medial septum (see also Fig. 1d and e).

We have observed that the time of initiation of ganglioside administration is crucial for the effective protection of forebrain cholinergic neurons. In young rats, when the initiation of ganglioside treatment was delayed for 10 days (30 mg/kg i.p. daily), no recovery in ChAT activity of the NBM was observed, even when administered for a total of 30 days. Based on these observations, we have administered the same dosage of GM_1 for 7 days starting from the first post-operative day and, in another series, commencing at the time of surgery. Only in the latter circumstance did ChAT enzymatic activity remain at control levels in the NBM following cortical lesions (Stephens et al., 1987). Therefore, with early commencement of treatment, short term administration of GM_1 resulted in an equally effective protection of cholinergic neurons from retrograde degeneration.

The possibility of reducing the amount of ganglioside required was also explored as this would enhance potential usefulness in larger animal models and future human clinical trials. Concurrently, we addressed the issue of a possible site of GM_1 action, i.e., peripheral vs. central. Effects of large (30 mg/kg) and small (5 mg/kg) doses of gangliosides on NBM cholinergic neurons were compared following decortication. Figure 2 summarizes these results which show that 5 mg/kg of GM_1 delivered intracerebroventricularly (i.c.v.) via osmotic minipumps, commencing at time of lesioning for only 7 days, rendered a biochemical protection of cholinergic neurons comparable to that of 30 mg/kg i.p. However, these small doses of ganglioside did not prevent cholinergic involution when applied systemically, suggesting a preferential central site of action. The short term i.c.v. administered GM_1 at the low dosage also conserved the morphology of ChAT immunoreactive NBM neurons as judged by quantitative image analysis.

It is worth noting that with the present therapeutic regimen (30 mg/kg i.p. daily for 30 days), GM_1 prevents retrograde degeneration of cholinergic NBM neurons in young

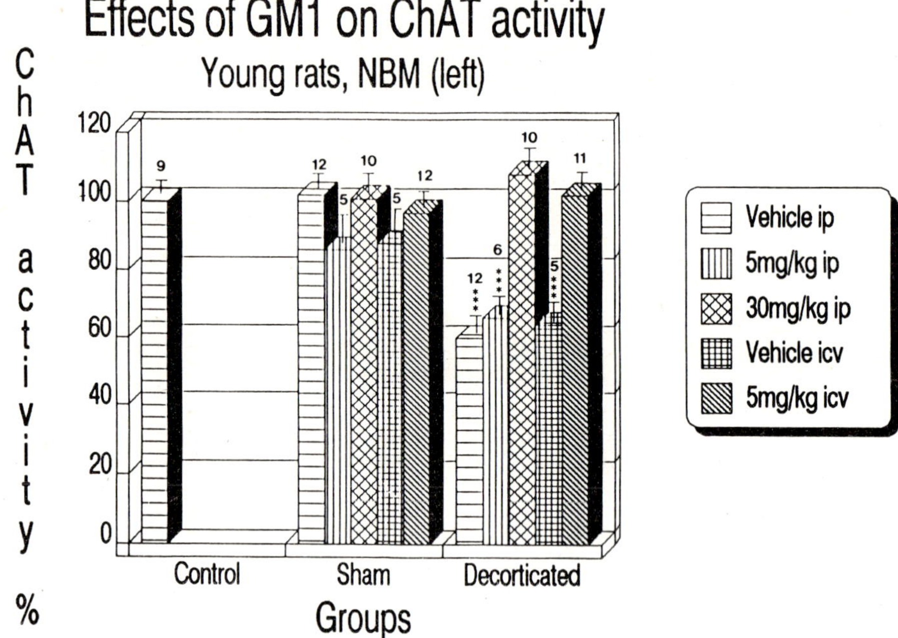

Figure 2. The effect of short-term GM$_1$ treatment initiated immediately following unilateral cortical lesion. Ganglioside GM$_1$ was administered intraperitoneally (i.p., 5 mg/kg (n = 6) or 30 mg/kg
(n = 10) daily for 7 days) or centrally (icv, 5 mg/kg (n = 11) by continuous infusion from osmotic
mini-pumps into the contralateral cerebral ventricle) commencing immediately after lesioning. Vehicle was administered ip (n = 12) or icv (n = 5) as above. Data were analysed by ANOVA and
Dunnett's test (***, p < 0.001) compared with the appropriate controls.

and mature rats but not in aged ones (2 years and older; Fig. 3). This lack of
responsiveness to GM$_1$ in the aged animal may be representative of the limited plastic
potential we have thus far observed in the older rat brain. Specifically, spontaneous
recovery of ChAT activity in the NBM of untreated young and mature animals but not
in aged rats occurs by 120 days after cortical lesioning (Fig. 4). Therefore, different
pharmacological approaches to overcome this limitation need to be explored since
application of these therapeutic strategies to the treatment of human neurodegenerative
conditions, most of which occur in the elderly, is inevitable.

Based on the aforementioned reports that NGF also influences cholinergic rat
forebrain neurons, it was important to compare the effects of GM$_1$ with those of NGF in
our cortex-basalis model of cholinergic retrograde degeneration. In this regard, our
results indicate that doses of NGF (i.c.v.) which produce stimulation of ChAT activity in
septo-hippocampal regions after partial transection of the fimbria (Hefti et al., 1984)
produce an analogous protection of the cholinergic neurons in the NBM. The
simultaneous administration of NGF and GM$_1$, however, resulted in a potentiation of
these effects. In these experiments the values of ChAT activity of the microdissected

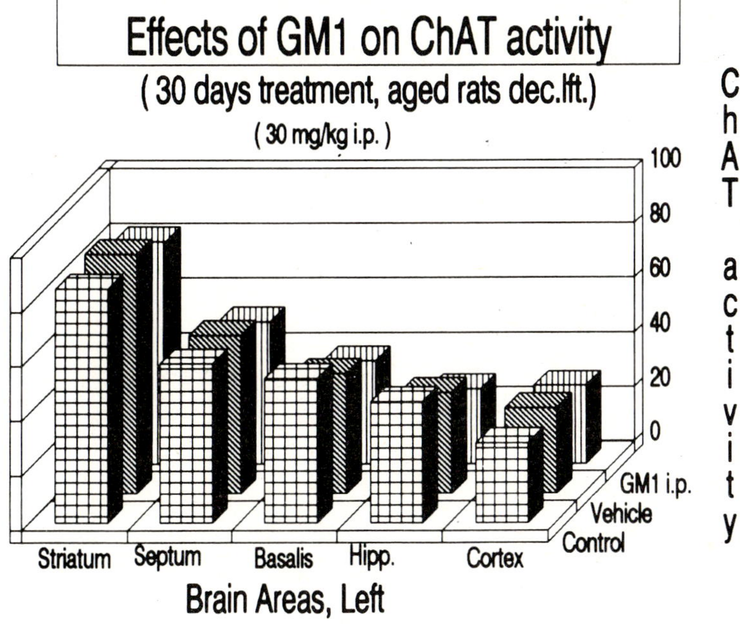

Figure 3. The effects of cortical lesions on ChAT activity in the NBM and other areas of the aged rat brain: chronic treatment with GM_1. Animals two years old at operation were unilaterally cortically lesioned and treated with vehicle or GM_1 i.p. (30 mg/kg intraperitoneally daily for 30 days). No changes were seen in ChAT activity (ordinate, nmols Ach/mg protein/hour) in any of the microdissected areas studied, except the NBM (basalis). Compared with sham-operated controls, a significant reduction (*, $p < 0.05$, unpaired t-test) in ChAT activity of the NBM was seen in both vehicle- and GM_1-treated animals.

NBM rose above normal in the lesioned side. Furthermore, in the remaining neocortex, ipsilateral to the lesion, ChAT activity rose to over 230% of control values (unpublished results).

EXPERIMENTAL EVIDENCE FOR A PROTECTIVE ROLE OF EMBRYONIC CORTICAL IMPLANTS ON FOREBRAIN CHOLINERGIC NEURONS

In addition to the aforementioned pharmacological approaches of protecting the cholinergic neurons in the NBM after cortical lesioning, we have recently transplanted embryonic rat cortical cells into the neocortex. Here we report preliminary results of successful cortical graft survival in devascularized cortex and at least partial prevention of retrograde neuronal degeneration in the ipsilateral NBM. This represents the first attempt at obtaining cortical cell survival in severely ischemic neocortex although an earlier study has shown protection of NBM cholinergic neurons after embryonic cortical cell implantation into kainic acid-lesioned cortex (Sofroniew et al., 1986b). In addition to identifying the cholinergic neurons of the nucleus with an anti-ChAT monoclonal antibody (Eckenstein and Thoenen, 1982), a monoclonal antibody against NGF receptor (NGFr) was also used (Chandler et al., 1984).

Neocortex of 3-month-old male Wistar rats was devascularized unilaterally in the usual manner by mechanically disrupting the surface pial blood vessels. Age and sex matched sham operated animals served as controls. A group of lesioned rats received six

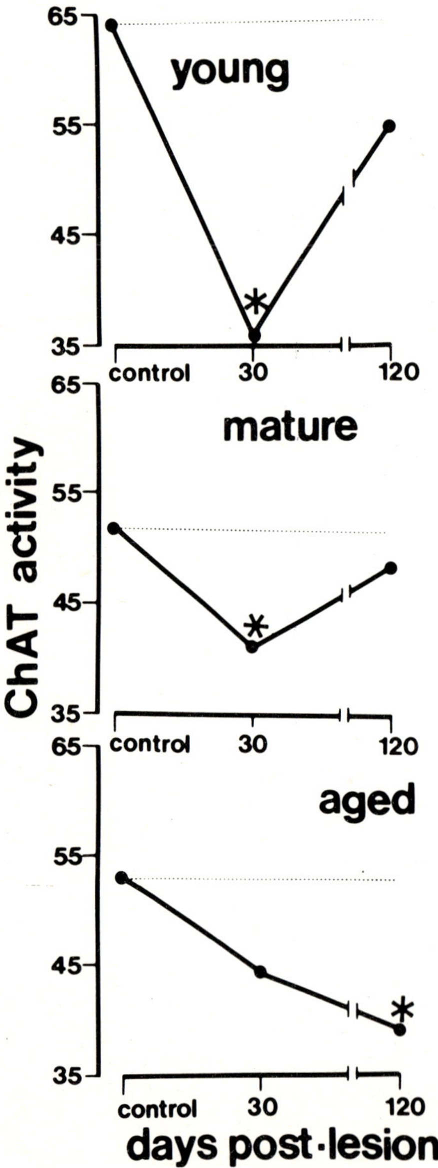

Figure 4. Retrograde biochemical effects on the ChAT activity of the microdissected ipsilateral nucleus basalis of the rat following unilateral cortical lesions in variously aged animals. ChAT activity (ordinate, nmols ACh/mg protein/hour) was significantly reduced (*, $p < 0.05$ compared with controls, n = 4-12) after lesions in all the age groups. A spontaneous recovery was noted in the young and mature animals (30 and 120 days old at operation), but not in the aged (2 years at surgery).

3 μl injections of cortical cell suspensions prepared from 16-17 gestational day Wistar rat embryo brains into the devascularized neocortex 6 days post-lesioning. Each injection contained approximately 8.1×10^4 viable cortical cells. Figure 4 summarizes the donor cell suspension preparation and injection procedure used (adapted from Björklund et al., 1983).

Our preliminary results suggest that in animals with significant survival and growth of cortical grafts, an apparent protective effect on NBM neurons occurs as demonstrated by ChAT and NGFr immunocytochemistry (Fig. 5). There is less neuronal and neurite shrinkage in the NBM of lesioned animals receiving implants than in those without grafts. This was particularly evident with the abundant plexus of NGFr immunoreactive neurites which these neurons displayed.

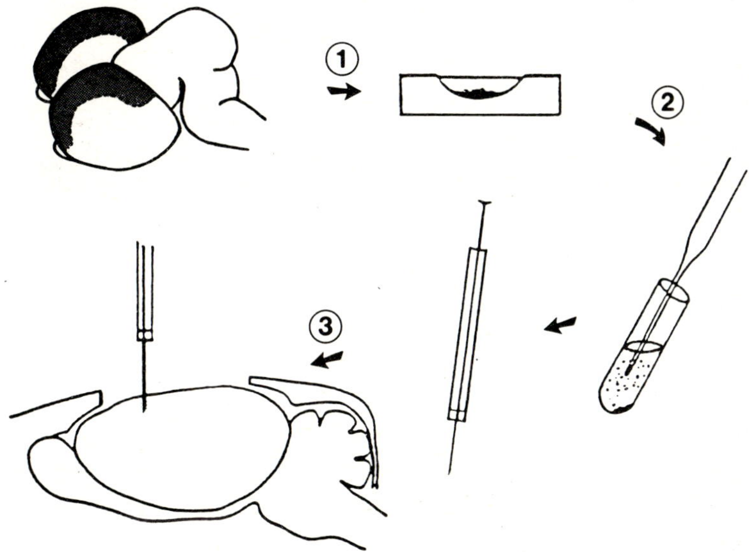

Figure 5. Diagrammatic representation of the preparation and implantation of embryonic cortical grafts (after Björklund et al., 1983). 1) Cortical tissue (shaded area) was dissected from rat embryo brains (embryonic day 16-17). 2) The tissue was trypsinized, washed, and a suspension of cortical cells obtained by mechanical dissociation. 3) The resulting preparation was injected at defined stereotaxic coordinates into the devascularised rat neocortex.

DISCUSSION

The present experimental model for retrograde degeneration of forebrain cholinergic neurons supports the hypothesis that the subcortical cholinergic involvement observed in Alzheimer's disease and related conditions might be caused by a primary cortical lesion. This view is also substantiated by evidence in Alzheimer brains of losses of cortical somatostatin immunoreactivity (Davies et al., 1980; Beal et al., 1986) which in the neocortex is apparently restricted to local circuit neurons and by the possible involvement of somatostatin immunoreactive neurons in early senile plaques (Morrison et al., 1985; Roberts et al., 1985). Assuming that the present experimental model parallels a retrograde deterioration of cholinergic forebrain neurons as may occur in Alzheimer's disease, it is of interest to investigate the possibilities of arresting or reversing such a process.

The particular responsiveness of CNS cholinergic neurons to GM_1 and NGF offers certain hopes that trophic factors might promote growth and repair of these neurons. In support of this, we have observed a remarkable recovery of the acetylcholine biosynthetic enzyme, ChAT, in the nucleus basalis as described above. Similar recoveries in biochemical parameters of cholinergic function have also been reported in the reverse situation, i.e. after stereotaxic lesions of the NBM (Wenk et al., 1984; Casamenti et al., 1985). In our retrograde degeneration model, this capacity for spontaneous recovery is absent in aged animals, which may be due to the apparent diminution of endogenous trophic factors in response to CNS injuries that has been observed in aged animals (Nieto-Sampedro et al., 1982). Gangliosides are also able to prevent the dramatic loss of cholinergic cell neurons subsequent to hippocampal ablation (Sofroniew et al., 1986a). A similar protection of septal cholinergic neurons following fimbria-fornix lesioning has been achieved using intracerebroventricular administration of NGF (Kromer, 1986; Hefti, 1986). The ability of gangliosides to prevent such cholinergic cell losses without exogenous NGF is remarkable since removal of the target site, i.e. hippocampus, has removed the major source of NGF which the septal neurons require for trophic effects. Gangliosides have similarly been shown to stimulate the re-innervation of the hippocampus after partial lesions of the fimbria (Oderfeld-Nowak et al., 1984), or septal nucleus (Wojcik et al., 1982).

We have demonstrated that the time of initiating ganglioside treatment, its duration and the total amount administered are relevant to the development of the therapeutic potential of GM_1. A delay of just one day with the low dose-short treatment scheme or a 10 day delay with the high dose-prolonged treatment protocol greatly attenuates ganglioside effectiveness. In contrast, small amounts of GM_1 are capable of preventing NBM degenerative changes when applied from the onset of cortical lesioning. The importance of early treatment with gangliosides concurs with the concept of a critical period of low availability of endogenous trophic factors immediately after lesions of the nervous system (Toffano et al., 1987). It is therefore conceivable that these observations all reflect neural responses to a balance between exogenously administered GM_1 and endogenous trophic factors. Such a proper balance is likely essential for securing the protection of neuronal elements after direct or indirect cellular distruption.

In the cortex-basalis retrograde degeneration model discussed here, a dissociation is observed between biochemical (ChAT activity) and morphological (cell size) parameters in the NBM of untreated young and mature rats 120 days after neocortical lesions (results not shown). A differential participation of multiple, uncharacterized endogenous factors could explain such a dissociation in these signs of recovery in young and mature animals. Evidence for the existence of separate factors regulating biochemical and morphological parameters in cholinergic neurons has been produced by Smith and collaborators (1983a; 1985b; 1986). There may, therefore, exist a variety of CNS trophic factors acting on subsets of transmitter-specific neurons and even on various aspects of an individual neuron's physiological functioning. Neurotrophic factors are apparently

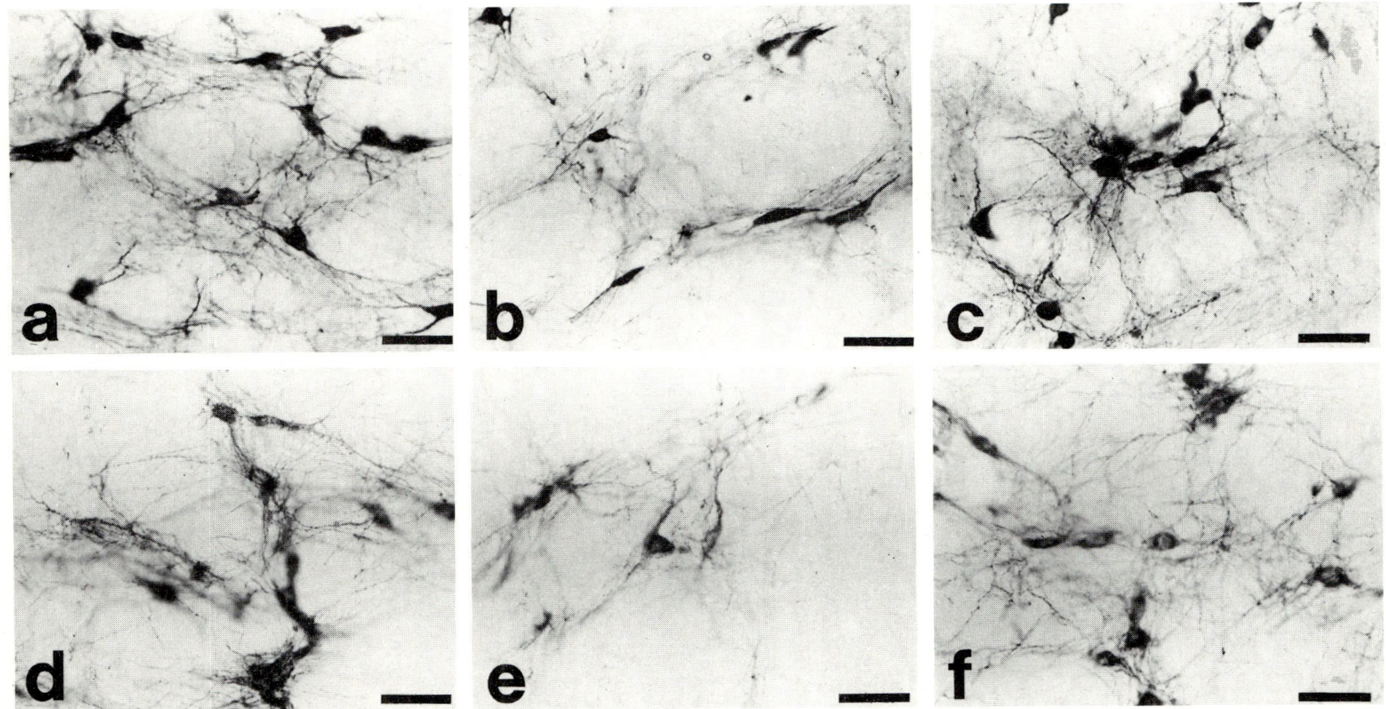

Figure 6. Inhibition of the retrograde morphological effects of cortical lesions on rat NBM ChAT and NGFr immunoreactive neurons. ChAT immunoreactivity was revealed (upper row) as described in the legend to Figure 1. NGFr immunoreactive elements were demonstrated in adjacent sections (lower row) using mouse monoclonal antibodies directed against NGFr (Chandler et al., 1984) and horseradish peroxidase (Semenenko et al., 1986). Left: In contralateral NBM from untreated cortically lesioned animals, ChAT (a) and NGFr (d) immunoreactive neurons display a normal appearance after 6 months. Centre: ChAT (b) and NGFr (e) immunopositive NBM cells present a shrunken appearance with loss of processes ipsilateral to the lesioned cortex. Right: In animals 6 months after cortical implants in the lesioned area of the cortex, cholinergic (c) and NGFr (f) somata on the lesioned side reveal a relatively normal appearance with abundant processes. Scale bar = 100 micrometres in all micrographs.

released when a CNS lesion occurs, the amount being dependent on the time after lesioning and the animal's age (Nieto-Sampedro et al., 1982). This is in line with our observations that the protective effects of GM_1 in the model of retrograde degeneration of cholinergic neurons are also dependent on the age of the recipient. Aside from their experimental relevance, these aspects, including age, dosage, initiation and duration of treatment, should be carefully considered in the possible development of ganglioside therapeutic strategies for the treatment of human neurodegenerative disorders, such as Alzheimer's disease.

The mechanisms by which gangliosides bring about these protective effects on cholinergic neurons are not yet understood. The cooperativity found in our studies with the simultaneous administration of GM_1 and NGF is suggestive of interactions with trophic factors. For example, GM_1 may facilitate the interactions between trophic factors and their corresponding membrane receptors. Membrane incorporation of exogenous gangliosides can occur in neuronal membrane preparations (Toffano et al., 1980) where they could thereby elicit a number of ligand-receptor interactions. Further knowledge of the nature of endogenous factors released as a consequence of neural injury and their receptors will provide a firmer base for the understanding of these cell membrane-ganglioside interactions.

The embryonic cortical cells implanted into lesioned rat neocortex of our model have been shown to at least partially reverse the retrograde degenerative changes of the ipsilateral cholinergic NBM neurons. Moreover, the rich plexus of NGFr immunoreactive neurites seen here suggests a sprouting phenomenon likely related to cortical transplant influences. In addition to replacing the anatomical projection site of these cholinergic neurons, the implanted donor tissue per se may be a source of various neurotrophic factors which contribute to graft survival in the ischemic milieu and possibly stimulate growth of surviving NBM nerve fibres. It is unclear, at present, to what degree potential trophic influences intrinsic to transplanted tissue may affect donor-host CNS interactions. Our future research in this direction will examine if exogenous ganglioside and NGF can enhance the effects of endogenous neurotrophic factors in cortically lesioned rats receiving transplants in order to achieve greater graft survival and more complete recovery of NBM neurons. The demonstration of significant neural protection in animal models using these therapeutic means is an important requirement before extending such treatment strategies to a clinical application in the human.

ACKNOWLEDGEMENTS

This work is dedicated to the inspiring and pioneering contributions of Professor Rita Levi-Montalcini. The authors acknowledge support from the Medical Research Council of Canada, Fidia Laboratories Spa (Abano Terme), Medicorp Inc (Montreal) and the Office of the Dean of the Faculty of Medicine, McGill University. Nerve growth factor was generously provided by Drs Levi-Montalcini and Aloe. Antibodies were generously provided against ChAT by Boehringer Mannheim (FDR) and against NGF receptor by E.M. Johnson. The secretarial assistance of Elaine Louw, and the photographic expertise of Alan Forster are gratefully appreciated.

REFERENCES

Appel SH (1981) A unifying hypothesis for the cause of amyotrophic lateral sclerosis, parkinsonism, and Alzheimer's disease. Ann Neurol 10:499-505.

Beal MF, Benoit R, Mazurek MF, Bird ED, Martin JB (1986) Somatostatin-28(1-12)-like immunoreactivity is reduced in Alzheimer's diseased cerebral cortex. Brain Res 368:380-383.

Björklund A, Steveni U, Schmidt RH, Dunnett SB, Gage FH (1983) Intracerebral grafting of neuronal cell suspensions. I. Introduction and general methods of preparation. Acta Physiol Scand Supp 522: 1-9.

Bowen DM, Allen SJ, Benton JS, Goodhart MJ, Haan EA, Palmer AM, Sims NR, Smith DDT, Spillane JA, Esiri MM, Neary D, Snowdon JB, Wilcock GK, Davison AN (1983) Biochemical assessment of serotonergic and cholinergic dysfunction and cerebral atrophy in Alzheimer's disease. J Neurochem 41:266-272.

Casamenti F, Bracco L, Bartolin L, Faper G (1985) Effects of ganglioside treatment in rats with a lesion of the cholinergic forebrain nuclei. Brain Res 338:45-52.

Chandler CE, Parsons LM, Hosang M, Shooter EM (1984) A monoclonal antibody modulates the interaction of nerve growth factor with PC12 cells. J Biol Chem 259:6882-6889.

Cuello AC, Sofroniew MV (1984) The anatomy of the CNS cholinergic neurons. Trends Neurosci 7:74-78.

Cuello AC, Milstein D, Wright B, Bramwell B, Priestley JV, Jarvis J (1984) Development and application of a monoclonal rat peroxidase anti-peroxidase (PAP) immunocytochemical reagent. Histochemistry 30:257-261.

Cuello AC, Stephens PH, Tagari PD, Sofroniew MV, Pearson RCA (1986) Retrograde changes in the nucleus basalis of the rat, caused by cortical damage, are prevented by exogenous ganglioside GM1. Brain Res 376:373-377.

Davies P, Maloney AJF (1976) Selective loss of central cholinergic neurons in Alzheimer's Disease. Lancet II:1403.

Davies P, Katzman R, Terry RD (1980) Reduced somatostatin like immunoreactivity in cerebral cortex of cases of Alzheimer's disease and Alzheimer's senile dementia. Nature 288:279-280.

Dunnett SB, Bjorklund A, Steveni U, Iversen SD (1981) Grafts of embryonic substantia nigra reinnervating the ventrolateral striatum ameliorate sensorimotor impairments and akinesia in rats with 6-OHDA lesions of the nigrostriatal pathway. Brain Res 229:209-217.

Eckenstein F, Thoenen H (1982) Production of specific antisera and monoclonal antibodies to choline acetyltransferase: characterization and use for identification of cholinergic neurons. EMBO J 1:363-368.

Fibiger HC (1982) The organization and some projections of cholinergic neurons of the mammalian forebrain. Brain Res Rev 4:327-388.

Gnahn H, Hefti F, Heumann R, Schwab ME (1983) NGF-mediated increase in choline acetyltransferase in the neonatal rat forebrain: evidence for a physiological role for NGF in the brain. Develop Brain Res 9:45-52.

Gorio A, Marini P, Zanoni R (1983) Muscle reinnervation - III. Motoneuron sprouting capacity, enhancement by exogenous gangliosides. Neuroscience 8(3):417-429.

Hefti F (1983) Alzheimer's disease caused by a lack of nerve growth factor? Ann Neurol 13:109-110.

Hefti F (1986) Nerve growth factor promotes survival of septal cholinergic neurons after fimbrial transections. J Neurosci 6:2155-2162.

Hefti F, Dravid A, Hartikka J (1984) Chronic intraventricular injections of nerve growth factor elevate hippocampal choline acetyltransferase activity in adult rats with partial septo-hippocampal lesions. Brain Res 293:305-311.

Hefti F, Hartikka J, Eckenstein F, Gnahn H, Heumann R, Schwab ME (1985) Nerve growth factor increases choline acetyltransferase but not survival or fibre outgrowth of cultured foetal septal cholinergic neurons. Neuroscience 14:55-68.

Honegger P, Lenior D (1983) Nerve growth factor (NGF) stimulation of cholinergic telencephalic neurons in aggregating cell cultures. Develop Brain Res 3:229-238.

Ingham CA, Bolam JP, Wainer BJ, Smith AD (1985) A correlated light and electron microscopic study of identified cholinergic basal forebrain neurons that project to the cortex in the rat. J Comp Neurol 239:176-192.

Johnston MV, McKinney M, Coyle JT (1981) Neocortical cholinergic innervation: a description of extrinsic and intrinsic components in the rat. Brain Res 43:159-172.

Karpiak SE (1983) Ganglioside treatment improves recovery of alteration behavior after unilateral entorhinal cortex lesion. Exp Neurol 81:330-339.

Korsching S (1986) The role of nerve growth factor in the CNS. Trends Neurosci 9:570-573.

Korsching S, Auburger G, Heumann R, Scott J, Thoenen H (1985) Levels of nerve growth factor and its mRNA in the central nervous system of the rat correlate with cholinergic innervation. EMBO J 4:1389-1393.

Kromer LF (1983) Utilization of neural transplants to analyze regeneration in the adult mammalian central nervous system. In: Wallace RB, Das GD (eds): Neural Tissue Transplantation Research. Springer-Verlag, New York, pp. 135-164.

Kromer LF (1986) Nerve growth factor treatment after brain injury prevents neuronal death. Science 235:214-216.

Lehman J, Nagy JI, Almadja S, Fibiger HC (1982) The nucleus basalis magnocellularis: the origin of a cholinergic projection to the neocortex in the rat. Neuroscience 5:1161-1174.

Levi-Montalcini R, Angeletti PU (1968) Nerve growth factor. Physiol Rev 48:534-569.

Lewis PR, Shute CCD (1967) The cholinergic limbic system: projections to hippocampal formation, medial cortex, nuclei of the ascending cholinergic reticular system and the subfornical organ and supra-optic crest. Brain 90:521-540.

Meibach RC, Siegel A (1977) Efferent connections of the hippocampal formation in the rat. Brain Res 124:197-224.

Mesulam M, Mufson EJ, Wainer BH (1986) Three-dimensional representation and cortical projection topography of the nucleus basalis (Ch4) in the macaque: concurrent demonstration of choline acetyltransferase and retrograde transport with a stabilised tetramethylbenzidine method for horseradish peroxidase. Brain Res 367:301-308.

Mobley WC, Rutowski JL, Tennekoon GI, Gemski J, Buchanan K, Johnston MV (1986) Nerve growth factor increases choline acetyltransferase activity in developing basal forebrain neurons. Mol Brain Res 1:53-62.

Morrison H, Rogers J, Scherr S, Benoit R, Bloom F (1985) Somatostatin activity in neuritic plaques. Nature 314:90-92.

Nieto-Sampedro M, Lewis ER, Cotman CW, Manthorpe EM, Skaper SD, Barbin G, Longo FM, Waron S (1982) Brain injury causes a time dependent increase in neuron trophic activity at the lesion site. Science 217:860-861.

Oblinger MM, Das GD (1983) Connectivity of transplants in the cerebellum: a model of developmental differences in neuroplasticity. In: Wallace RB, Das GD (eds): Neural Tissue Transplantation Research. Springer-Verlag, New York, pp. 105-133.

Oderfeld-Nowak B, Narkiewicz O, Bialowas J, Wieraszko A, Gradkowska M (1974) The influence of septal nuclei lesions on activity of acetylcholinesterase and choline acetyltransferase in the hippocampus of the rat. Acta Neurobiol Exp 34:583-601.

Oderfeld-Nowak B, Skup M, Ulas J, Jezierska M, Gradkowska R, Zaremba M (1984) Effect of GM_1 ganglioside treatment on post lesion responses of cholinergic neurons in rat hippocampus after various partial deafferentiations. J Neurosci Res 12:409-420.

Perry EK, Tomlinson BE, Blessed G, Bergmann K, Gibson PH, Perry RH (1978) Correlation of cholinergic abnormalities with senile plaques and mental stress in senile dementia. Brit Med J II:1457-1459.

Raivich G, Kreutzberg GW (1987) The localization and distribution of high affinity beta-nerve growth factor binding sites in the central nervous system of the adult rat. A light microscopic autoradiographic study using (^{125}I)beta-nerve growth factor. Neuroscience 20:23-36.

Richardson PM, Verge Issa VMK, Riopelle RJ (1986) Distribution of neuronal receptors for nerve growth factor in the rat. J Neurosci 6:2312-2321.

Roberts GW, Crow TJ, Polak JM (1985) Location of neuronal tangles in somatostatin neurons in Alzheimer's disease. Nature 314:92-94.

Rossor MN, Svendsen C, Hunt SF, Mountjoy CG, Roth M, Iversen LL (1982) The substantia innominata in Alzheimer's disease: a histochemical and biochemical study of cholinergic marker enzymes. Neurosci Lett 28:217-222.

Schwab ME, Otten U, Agid Y, Thoenen H (1979) Nerve growth factor (NGF) in the rat CNS: absence of specific retrograde axonal transport and tyrosine hydroxylase induction in locus coeruleus and substantia nigra. Brain Res 168:473-483.

Seiler M, Schwab ME (1984) Specific retrograde transport of nerve growth factor (NGF) from neocortex to nucleus basalis in the rat. Brain Res 300:33-39.

Semenenko FM, Bramwell S, Sidebottom E, Cuello AC (1986) Development of a mouse anti-peroxidase secreting hybridoma for use in the production of a mouse PAP complex for immunocytochemistry and as a parent line in the development of hybrid hybridomas. Histochemistry 83:405-408.

Sims NR, Bowen DM, Allan SJ, Smith CCT, Neary D, Thomay DJ, Davison AN (1983) Presynaptic cholinergic dysfunction in patients with dementia. J Neurochem 401:503-509.

Smith RG, Appel SH (1983a) Extracts of skeletal muscle increase neurite outgrowth and cholinergic activity of foetal rat spinal motor neurons. Science 219:1079-1081.

Smith RG, McNaman RJ, Appel SH (1983b) Trophic effects of skeletal muscle extracts on ventral spinal cord neurons: in vitro separation of a protein with morphologic activity from proteins with cholinergic activity. J Cell Biol 101:1608-1621.

Smith RG, Vaca K, McNaman J, Appel SH (1986) Selective effects of skeletal muscle extract fractions on motorneuron development in vitro. J Neurosci 6:439-447.

Sofroniew MV, Eckenstein F, Thoenen H, Cuello AC (1983a) Topography of choline acetyltransferase-containing neurons in the forebrain of the rat. Neurosci Lett 33:7-12.

Sofroniew MV, Pearson RCA, Eckenstein F, Cuello AC, Powell TPS (1983b) Retrograde changes in cholinergic neurons in the basal forebrain of the rat following cortical damage. Brain Res 289:370-374.

Sofroniew MV, Pearson RCA, Cuello AC, Tagari PC, Stephens PM (1986a) Parenterally administered GM$_1$ ganglioside prevents retrograde degeneration of cholinergic cells of the rat basal forebrain. Brain Res 398:393-396.

Sofroniew MV, Isacson O, Bjorklund A (1986b) Cortical grafts prevent atrophy of cholinergic basal nucleus neurons induced by excitotoxic cortical damage. Brain Res 378:409-415.

Stephens PH, Cuello AC, Sofroniew MV, Pearson RDA, Tagari P (1985) The effect of unilateral decortication upon choline acetyltransferase and glutamate decarboxylase activities in the nucleus basalis and other areas of the rat brain. J Neurochem 45:1021-1026.

Stephens PH, Tagari PC, Garofalo L, Maysinger D, Piotte M, Cuello AC (1987) Neural plasticity of basal forebrain cholinergic neurons: effects of gangliosides. Neurosci Lett 80:80-84.

Taniuchi M, Schweitzer JB, Johnson EM (1986) Nerve growth factor receptor molecules in rat brain. Proc Nat Acad Sci USA 83:1950-1954.

Toffano G, Benvegnu D, Bonetti A, Facci L, Leon A, Orlando F, Ghidoni R, Tettamanil G (1980) Interaction of GM$_1$ ganglioside with crude rat brain neuronal membranes. J Neurochem 35:861-866.

Toffano G, Dal Toso R, Facci L, Ferrari G, Benvegnú D, Consolazione A, Favaron M, Leon A (1987) Gangliosides as Modulators of Neuronotrophic Interactions. In: Fuxe K, Agnati L (eds): Receptor-Receptor Interactions. Wenner-Gren International Symposium Series. Vol. 48, the Macmillan Press Ltd, London, pp. 54-61.

Wenk GL, Olton DS (1984) Recovery of neocortical ChAT activity following ibotenic acid injection into the nucleus basalis of Meynert in rats. Brain Res 293:184-186.

Whitehouse PJ, Price DL, Struble RG, Clark AW, Coyle JT, DeLong MR (1982) Alzheimer's disease and senile dementia loss of neurons in the basal forebrain. Science 215:1237-1239.

Wojcik M, Ules J, Oderfeld-Nowak B (1982) The stimulating effect of ganglioside injections on the recovery of choline acetyltransferase and acetylcholinesterase activities in the hippocampus of the rat after septal lesions. Neuroscience 7:495-499.

Neuronal Plasticity and Trophic Factors
G. Biggio, P.F. Spano, G. Toffano, S.H. Appel, G.L. Gessa (eds.)
Fidia Research Series, Symposia in Neuroscience VII
Liviana Press, Padova © 1988

EFFECTS OF PERIPHERAL NERVE GRAFTS ON THE SURVIVAL AND REGROWTH OF AXOTOMIZED CNS NEURONS

Garth M. Bray, Maria Paz Villegas-Pérez, Manuel Vidal-Sanz and Albert J. Aguayo

Neurosciences Unit, The Montreal General Hospital and McGill University, 1650 Cedar Avenue, Montréal, H3G 1A4, Québec, Canada

INTRODUCTION

In adult mammals, extensive axonal regrowth and terminal reconnectivity are limited to certain types of injury in the peripheral nervous system. Following crush injury of a peripheral nerve, there can be a nearly complete restoration of nerve fiber structure (Cragg and Thomas, 1964; Devor and Govrin-Lippmann, 1979; Diamond and Jackson, 1980) and function (Burgess and Horch, 1973; Burgess et al., 1974; Dykes and Terzis, 1979); because Schwann cell basal laminas are not extensively disrupted by this type of injury, many columns of Schwann cells remain aligned to direct the regenerating axons to their appropriate targets. After complete transection of peripheral nerves (PN), however, many axons fail to reach their specific targets because of the misalignment of the Schwann cells columns disrupted at the site of injury, and functional recovery is incomplete (Horch and Burgess, 1980), in spite of surgical apposition of the proximal and distal nerve stumps.

CNS neurons are also able to elongate their injured axons and restore connectivity and function in certain amphibians and fish. If the optic nerves (ON) are transected in the adult goldfish, for example, retinal ganglion cells survive, regenerate their axons, and reform synapses in the optic tectum with a restoration of visual function (for a review, see Grafstein, 1986). In adult mammals, on the other hand, interruption of the optic nerve or other CNS pathways leads to abortive axonal sprouting without axonal elongation so that target neurons remain permanently disconnected.

Experimental Enhancement of the Regeneration of CNS Axons in Adult Mammals

Local axonal growth for distances of a few millimeters has been observed after small injuries near cell bodies in the retina (Leoz and Arcaute, 1914; Goldberg and Frank, 1980; McConnell and Berry, 1982; So et al., 1986) or spinal cord (Risling et al., 1983; Havton and Kellerth, 1987). Furthermore, the introduction of fetal neural tissues or iridis into the CNS (Bjorklund and Stenevi, 1984) has provided evidence of the responsiveness of mature central neurons to targets in their immediate environment. But neither the sprouts of nerve cells indigenous to the adult host CNS nor those arising from transplanted fetal neurons have elongated successfully for the distances necessary to restore major projections in the brain and spinal cord, an indication that substrate conditions within the mature CNS of mammals either fail to promote substantial elongation or exert inhibitory effects on neurite extension.

There is, however, an expanding body of experimental evidence which indicates that the regenerative responses of axotomized CNS neurons in adult mammals can be modified by external influences (for a review, see Aguayo, 1985). Based on light microscopic studies early in this century, Ramón y Cajal (1914) recognized that CNS axons in adult mammals would grow into peripheral nerve segments. With the application of intraaxonally-transported tracer substances, it was subsequently possible to establish that neurons in many parts of the CNS can elongate their axons into PN grafts for several centimeters, distances even greater than those accomplished during normal development in the intact animal (David and Aguayo, 1981; Benfey and Aguayo, 1982; So and Aguayo, 1985; Vidal-Sanz et al., 1985; So et al., 1986). Such results indicate that, as suggested by Ramón y Cajal (1914), the non-neuronal components of peripheral nerve contain growth promoting properties that are lacking in the CNS milieu. Moreover, when PN grafts containing axons regenerating from the transected optic nerves of adult rats were inserted into the denervated superior colliculi, some synaptic connections were reformed (Vidal-Sanz et al., 1986; 1987). Thus, to a limited extent, the PN graft-induced changes in the environment of the growth cones of the interrupted axons have permitted these CNS neurons in adult mammals to replicate some of the processes that characterize the formation of neuronal circuitries during development as well as the reconstitution of certain injured CNS pathways in amphibians and fish.

The PN transplantation experiments also provided evidence that only axotomized neurons are responsive to the growth stimulating environment provided by the PN graft. Using retrograde labelling with two different fluorescent tracers, no evidence was obtained to suggest that axons from uninjured neurons had grown into grafts inserted into the retina (So and Aguayo, 1985) or the olfactory bulb (Friedman and Aguayo, 1985). Furthermore, greater numbers of CNS neurons grew their axons into PN grafts when the axotomy was close to the cell body than when it was located more distally (Richardson et al., 1984; Sceats et al., 1986).

Axotomy can also lead to a spectrum of retrograde changes that range from chromatolysis to the death of the injured neurons, particularly if the lesion is near the cell body (Lieberman, 1974). Thus, it was important to determine the effect of PN graft placement on the survival and regrowth of CNS neurons. Because the retina contains a well-characterized population of neurons whose arrangement is particularly suited for anatomical, functional, and molecular studies of the CNS regenerative capacities, we

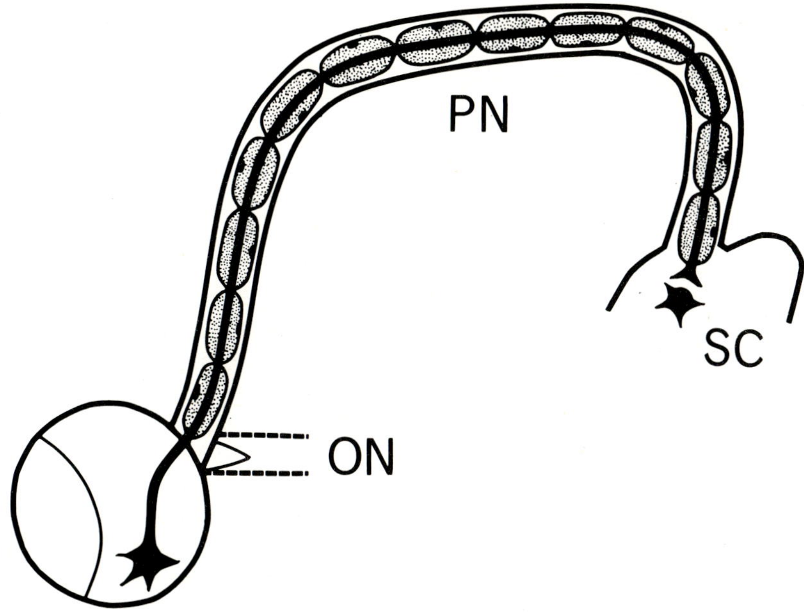

Figure 1. Diagram depicting an autologous peripheral nerve graft (PN) implanted between the eye and the superior colliculus (SC) to substitute for the totally transected optic nerve (ON) in an adult rat. Transected retinal ganglion cell axons grown into the graft, become ensheathed by Schwann cells and elongate along the length of the graft. When these axons reach the SC, their growth within the CNS is limited to less than one millimeter. (Reproduced from Bray et al., 1987 with permission of the Company of Biologists Limited).

used a series of adult Sprague-Dawley rats in which the ON was transected and replaced with an autologous segment of peroneal nerve (Fig. 1; Vidal-Sanz et al., 1985) to investigate the survival of retinal ganglion cells RGCs as well as the proportions of these surviving neurons that regrow their axons into the PN grafts. For these studies, axotomized ganglion cells in retinas with and without PN-grafts were examined by morphometric techniques, double-labelling with retrogradely-transported fluorescent markers, and immunological markers.

Effects of PN Grafts on Retinal Ganglion Cell Survival and Axonal Regrowth

It was previously demonstrated that axotomized RGCs share with other CNS neurons a capacity to regenerate axons for distances of 1-3 cm into PN grafts that were either inserted directly into the retinas of adult rats (So and Aguayo, 1985) or attached to the ocular stumps of optic nerves (ON) transected near the retina (Vidal-Sanz et al., 1985; 1987). Furthermore, some of these retinal neurons that have elongated their axons into the PN grafts showed apparently normal electrophysiologic responses to ocular stimulation by light (Keirstead et al., 1985).

124

Retinal Ganglion Cell Survival after Axotomy and PN Grafting

Approximately one-half of the neurons in the ganglion cell layer of the retinas of adult rodents die after axotomy (Grafstein and Ingoglia, 1982; Misantone et al., 1984; Allcutt et al., 1984; Berry et al., 1986; Villegas-Pérez et al., 1986; 1988). However, assessments of cell death based only on counts of the total numbers of surviving neurons in the ganglion cell layer do not distinguish between the actual ganglion cells and the many axonless amacrine cells present in this layer (Perry, 1981; Linden and Perry, 1983). Moreover, estimates based on size criteria alone are relatively inaccurate because of the overlap between large amacrine cells and small RGCs (Perry, 1981). Thus, we used 1,1'-Dioctadecyl-3,3,3',3'-tetramethylindocarbocyanine (diI), a retrogradely transported tracer that remains in neurons for long periods of time (Honig and Hume, 1986) to estimate the densities of surviving RGCs in axotomized and PN-grafted retinas (Villegas-Pérez et al., 1986; 1988). Examined from 15 days to 3 months after axotomy, the densities of surviving RGCs in the retinas of these animals were two to four-fold greater in the retinas with PN grafts (Fig. 2). In retinas examined after longer intervals (6 and 9 months), the effects of PN grafts were assessed by identifying intra-retinal RGC axons by their immunoreactivity to RT 97, a monoclonal antibody to 200 kDa subunits of the neurofilaments (Anderton et al., 1982). In such preparations, there was a striking

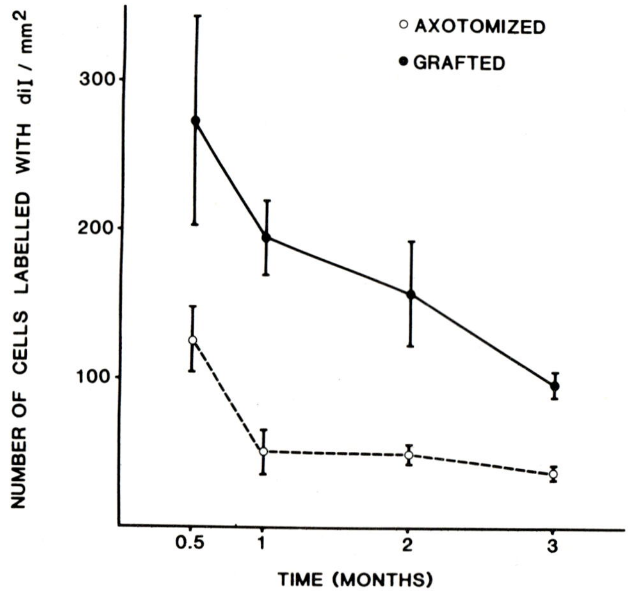

Figure 2. Mean densities ($\pm$S.E.M.) of retinal ganglion cells (RGCs) labelled with the retrogradely-transported tracer, diI, applied to the optic nerves at the time of their transection near the eye. A peripheral nerve graft was attached to the ocular stump of one optic nerve in each animal. Two animals were examined at 15 days, 6 at 1 month, 4 at 2 months, and 6 at 3 months. At 1, 2, and 3 months, the differences in the denstities of surviving RGCs were significantly greater ($p<0.05$) after axotomy and PN grafting than after axotomy alone (Reproduced with permission from Villegas-Pérez et al., 1988).

enhancement of RCG axon preservation in the PN grafted retinas (Villegas-Pérez et al., 1988).

Axonal Regrowth by Surviving Retinal Ganglion Cells

In experiments in which two different fluorescent tracers were used to estimate the relative extents of survival and regrowth, it was found that as many as 20% of the surviving RGCs had grown their axons to the end of the PN grafts (Villegas-Pérez et al., 1986; 1988). Because not all re-growing axons may have reached the site of application of these tracers to the end of the grafts and some may not have incorporated the tracers used for these studies, the incidence of axonal regeneration among surviving RGCs may be even higher.

These results imply that early interactions between RGCs and the PN grafts mitigate the retrograde effects of axotomy on some of these retinal neurons by inducing the mature RGCs to mount the metabolic responses to axotomy that permit them to survive injury and to regrow lengthy axons. Although several mechanisms could be postulated to explain these effects, it is possible that neuronal survival may not necessarily require retinal axonal extension into the grafts but may be mediated by molecules released by graft components acting on RGCs soon after injury (Villegas-Pérez et al., 1988).

COMMENTS

Effective regeneration after axotomy depends on:
— survival of the axotomized neurons;
— axonal growth by the sprouting of axons from the proximal nerve stumps and their subsequent elongation and guidance to proper targets;
— axonal ensheathment and differentiation;
— the re-establishment of connectivity through synaptic contacts with target cells;
— the loss of inappropriate connections or redundant axon branches; and
— the maintenance of these regenerated connections in a functional, adaptable state. Although some of our results indicated that grafted segments of peripheral nerve can enhance the survival of the axotomized neurons, promote and guide the elongation of their axons, and permit the formation of new synapses, several questions need to be explored before it can be suggested that the axonal regeneration in adult mammals can lead to a restoration of neuronal circuitry.

Without experimental manipulations such as the use of PN grafts, the CNS environment that surrounds injured axons appears to provide little support for the survival of axotomized neurons. In the experiments of Villegas-Pérez et al. (1986; 1988), nearly 90% of all RGCs died soon after cutting the ON; a similar loss has been reported in adult rats among the cholinergic neurons of the nucleus basalis following the sectioning of the fimbria-fornix (Hefti, 1986; Williams et al., 1986; Kromer, 1987). However, although conditions in the injured CNS did not substantially protect either of these populations of neurons from undergoing retrograde degeneration in response to axotomy, their survival was enhanced by experimentally applied external influences –

126

PN grafts in the case of the axotomized RGCs (Villegas-Pérez et al., 1988) and Nerve Growth Factor (NGF) in the case of the cholinergic nucleus basalis neurons (Hefti, 1986; Williams et al., 1986; Kromer, 1987). In other words, these neurons have proven capable of overcoming some of the effects of injury when they were provided with critical trophic molecules or tissues that presumably contain molecules, as yet unidentified, with analogous effects.

Although PN grafts appear to enhance the early survival of axotomized neurons, there is experimental evidence to suggest that the viability of regenerating neurons that are prevented from forming terminal connections may not be sustained indefinitely by the contact of their axons with the non-neuronal environment of peripheral nerve. In the PN-grafted retinas examined 9 and 12 months after axotomy, the course of many of the surviving RGC axons became distorted and irregular (Vidal-Sanz, Villegas-Pérez, Bray and Aguayo, unpublished observations) and there was a progressive loss of their cells of origin (Villegas-Pérez et al., 1988). Furthermore, axons that had regenerated into PN grafts from the retina (Keirstead et al., 1985) or the brainstem of adult rats (Gauthier and Rasminsky, 1988) have shown decreasing responsiveness to physiological stimuli after periods of several months. Finally, when neurons from the fetal neopallium were transplanted into peripheral nerves of adult rats and isolated from their connections with the rest of the CNS, they undergo protracted cytoskeletal changes (Doering and Aguayo, 1987) that resemble those observed in the brains of aging animals. It remains an important objective to determine if such late morphological and functional effects on axotomized/PN grafted neurons can be prevented by the application of specific molecules or by the establishment of synaptic contacts with the target tissues to which they are guided.

Our working hypothesis has been that the elongation and guidance of axons to their targets, accomplished by the use of the PN grafts (Vidal-Sanz et al., 1987), could permit recognition phenomena that determine selective synaptogenesis. However, there is so far no evidence that such essential processes can be replicated in adult mammals. Because retinal projections are retinotopically arranged, it may be now possible to explore this question further in animals with PN bridges joining the eye and the superior colliculus. Furthermore, because one of the circumstances that has limited further studies of the connectivity and function of regenerated central axons is the fact that relatively few neurons extend along the PN bridges and re-enter the CNS (David and Aguayo, 1981; Vidal-Sanz et al., 1987), the present studies provide a clear indication for the need to develop strategies aimed specifically at increasing the viability of injured neurons as a potential source of regenerated axons that may reinnervate their targets.

ACKNOWLEDGEMENTS

The authors thank M. David, S. Harrington, J. Laganière, S. Shinn, J. Trecarten and W. Wilcox for technical assistance. M.P. V.-P. was supported by the Spanish Ministry of Education and Science. M. V.-S. was supported by the Luis Manuel Foundation and the Medical Research Council of Canada. The Medical Research Council, the Multiple Sclerosis Society, and the F.C.A.R. of Québec provided research grants.

REFERENCES

Aguayo AJ (1985) Axonal regeneration from injured neurons in the adult mammalian central nervous system. In: Cotman CW (ed): Synaptic Plasticity. Guilford Press, New York, pp. 457-484.

Allcutt D, Berry M, Sievers J (1984) A quantitative comparison of the reactions of retinal ganglion cells to optic nerve crush in neonatal and adult mice. Dev Brain Res 16: 219-230.

Anderton BH, Downes MJ, Green PJ, Tomlinson BE, Ulrich J, Wood JN, Kahn J (1982) Monoclonal antibodies show that neurofibrillary tangles and neurofilaments share antigenic determinants. Nature 298: 84-86.

Benfey M, Aguayo AJ (1982) Extensive elongation of axons from rat brain into peripheral nerve grafts. Nature 296: 150-152.

Berry M, Rees L, Sievers J (1986) Unequivocal regeneration of rat optic nerve axons into sciatic nerve isografts. In: Das GD, Wallace RB (eds): Neural Transplantation and Regeneration. Springer-Verlag, New York, pp. 63-79.

Bjorklund A, Stenevi U (1984) Intracerebral neural implants: neuronal replacement and reconstruction of damaged circuitries. Ann Rev Neurosci 7: 279-308.

Bray GM, Villegas-Pérez MP, Vidal-Sanz M, Aguayo AJ (1987) The use of peripheral nerve grafts to enhance neuronal survival, promote growth, and permit terminal reconnections in the central nervous system of adult rats. J Exp Biol 132:5-19.

Burgess PR, English KB, Horch KW, Stensaas LJ (1974) Patterning in the regeneration of type I cutaneous receptors. J Physiol (Lond) 236: 57-82.

Burgess PR, Horch KW (1973) Specific regeneration of cutaneous fibres in the cat. J Neurophysiol 36: 101-114.

Cragg BG, Thomas PK (1964) The conduction velocity of regenerating peripheral nerve fibres. J Physiol (Lond) 171:164-175.

David S, Aguayo AJ (1981) Axonal elongation into PNS "bridges" after CNS injury in adult rats. Science 214:931-933.

Devor M, Govrin-Lippmann R (1979) Selective regeneration of sensory nerve fibers following nerve crush injury. Exp Neurol 65: 243-254.

Diamond J, Jackson PC (1980) Regeneration and collateral sprouting of peripheral nerves. In: Jewett DL, McCarroll Jr HR (eds): Nerve Repair and Regeneration. Mosby, St Louis, pp. 115-127.

Doering L, Aguayo AJ (1987) Hirano bodies and other cytoskeletal abnormalities develop in fetal rat CNS grafts isolated for long periods in peripheral nerve. Brain Res 401: 178-184.

Dykes RW, Terzis JK (1979) Reinnervation of glabrous skin in baboons: Properties of cutaneous mechanoreceptors subsequent to nerve crush. J Neurophysiol 42: 461-478.

Friedman B, Aguayo AJ (1985) Injured neurons in the olfactory bulb of the adult rat grow new axons along peripheral nerve grafts. J Neurosci 5: 1616-1625.

Gauthier P, Rasminsky M (1988) Activity of medullary respiratory neurons regenerating axons into peripheral nerve grafts in the adult rat. Brain Res 438:225-236.

Goldberg S, Frank B (1980) Will the central nervous system in the adult mammal regenerate after bypassing a lesion? A study in the mouse and chick visual systems. Exp Neurol 70:675-689.

Grafstein B (1986) Regeneration in ganglion cells. In: Adler R, Farber D, (eds): The Retina. Academic Press, Orlando, Florida, pp. 275-335.

Grafstein B, Ingoglia NA (1982) Intracranial transection of the optic nerve in adult mice: Preliminary observations. Exp Neurol 76: 318-330.

Havton L, Kellerth J-O (1987) Regeneration by supernumerary axons with synaptic terminals in spinal motoneurons of cats. Nature 325: 711-714.

Hefti F (1986) Nerve growth factor promotes survival of septal cholinergic neurons after fimbrial transections. J Neurosci 6:2155-2162.

Honig MG, Hume RI (1986) Fluorescent carbocyanine dyes allow living neurons of identified origin to be studied in long-term cultures. J Cell Biol 103:171-187.

Horch KW, Burgess PR (1980) Functional specificity and somatotopic organization during peripheral nerve regeneration. In: Jewett DL, McCarroll Jr HR (eds): Nerve Repair and Regeneration. Mosby, St. Louis, Missouri, pp. 105-114.

Keirstead SA, Vidal-Sanz M, Rasminsky M, Aguayo AJ, Levesque M, So K-F (1985). Responses to light of retinal neurons regenerating axons into peripheral nerve grafts in the rat. Brain Res 359: 402-406.

Kromer LF (1987) Nerve growth factor treatment after brain injury prevents neuronal death. Science 235: 214-216.

Leoz Ortin G, Arcaute LR (1914) Procesos regenerativos del nervio optico y retina con ocasión de injertos nerviosos. Trab del Lab de Invest Biol 11: 239-254.

Lieberman AR (1974) Some factors affecting retrograde neuronal responses to axonal lesions. In: Bellairs R, Gray EG (eds): Essays of the Nervous System. Clarendon, Oxford, pp. 71-105.

McConnell P, Berry M (1982) Regeneration of axons in the mouse retina after injury. Bibl Anat 23: 26-37.

Misantone LJ, Gershenbaum M, Murray M (1984) Viability of retinal ganglion cells after optic nerve crush in adult rats. J Neurocytol 13: 449-465.

Perry VH (1981) Evidence for an amarcine cell system in the ganglion cell layer of the rat retina. Neuroscience 6: 931-944.

Ramón y Cajal S (1914) Degeneración y regeneración traumáticas en el nervio óptico y retina. In: Estudios sobre la degeneración y regeneración del sistema nervioso, T II. Imprenta de Hijos de Nicolás Moya, Madrid, Spain, pp. 203-217.

Richardson PM, Issa VMK, Aguayo AJ (1984) Regeneration of long spinal axons in the rat. J Neurocytol 13: 165-182.

Risling M, Cullheim S, Hildebrand C (1983) Reinnervation of the ventral root L7 from ventral horn neurons following intramedullary axotomy in adult rats. Brain Res 280: 15-23.

Sceats DJ, Friedman WA, Sypert GW, Ballinger WE (1986) Regeneration in peripheral nerve grafts to the cat spinal cord. Brain Res 362: 149-156.

So K-F, Aguayo AJ (1985) Lengthy regrowth of cut axons from ganglion cells after peripheral nerve transplantation into the retina of adult rats. Brain Res 328: 349-354.

So K-F, Xiao Y-M, Diao Y-C (1986) Effects on the growth of damaged ganglion cell axons after peripheral nerve transplantation in adult hamsters. Brain Res 377: 168-172.

Vidal-Sanz M, Villegas-Pérez MP, Cochard P, Aguayo AJ (1985) Axonal regeneration from the rat retina after total replacement of the optic nerve by a PNS graft. Soc Neurosci Abstr 11: 254.

Vidal-Sanz M, Bray GM, Aguayo AJ (1986) Terminal growth of regenerating retinal axons directed along PNS grafts to enter the midbrain in adult rats. Soc Neurosci Abst 12: 700.

Vidal-Sanz M, Bray GM, Villegas-Pérez MP, Thanos S, Aguayo AJ (1987) Axonal regeneration and synapse formation in the superior colliculus by retinal ganglion cells in the adult rat. J Neurosci 7:2894-2909.

Villegas-Pérez MP, Vidal-Sanz M, Aguayo AJ (1986) Effects of axotomy and PN grafting on adult rat retinal ganglion cells. Soc Neurosci Abstr 12: 700.

Villegas-Pérez MP, Vidal-Sanz M, Bray GM, Aguayo AJ (1988) Influence of peripheral nerve grafts on the survival and regrowth of axotomized retinal ganglion cells in the adult rat. J Neurosci 8:265-280.

Williams LR, Varon S, Peterson GM, Victorin K, Fisher W, Bjorklund A, Gage FH (1986) Continuous infusion of nerve growth factor prevents basal forebrain neuronal death after fimbria fornix transection. Proc Natl Acad Sci USA 83: 9231-9235.

Neuronal Plasticity and Trophic Factors
G. Biggio, P.F. Spano, G. Toffano, S.H. Appel, G.L. Gessa (eds.)
Fidia Research Series, Symposia in Neuroscience VII
Liviana Press, Padova © 1988

MECHANISMS OF PLASTICITY IN SHORT AND LONG TERM LEARNING PROCESSES IN INVERTEBRATES

M. Brunelli, L. Colombaioni and G. Traina

Department of Physiology and Biochemistry, University of Pisa
Via S. Zeno 31, 56100 Pisa, Italy

INTRODUCTION

The invertebrate nervous system has proved to be a useful model for the analysis of cellular and molecular mechanisms underlying short and long term behavioral modifications.

Studies performed on the invertebrate ganglia have yielded clear data on the events underlying simple forms of non-associative learning, such as habituation and sensitization. Parallel studies at the behavioral and cellular level have also been possible because the neuronal networks correlated with behavior and learning have been extensively described.

Taking as a behavioral model the gill and siphon withdrawal reflex in the marine mollusc *Aplysia*, Kandel demonstrated that the elementary synaptic connection between sensory and motor neurons changes in efficacy during simple forms of non-associative learning, such as habituation and sensitization. During habituation, the transmitter output from sensory neurons decreases.

Detailed information is also available on sensitization, a form of learning in which a test stimulus is potentiated when a strong noxious stimulus has been applied. This sensitizing stimulus triggers the release of substances acting on sensory neurons, thereby inducing a chain of events which, through the activation of an adenylate cyclase and the increase in the endogenous level of cAMP, leads to a cAMP-dependent protein phosphorylation which, in turn, promotes the closure of specific K channels (Ks).

The outward currents contributing to the repolarization of the sensory neuron action potential are thereby reduced causing an increase in the duration of the action potential which enhances the Ca^{++} influx and therefore the transmitter release. This mechanism of heterosynaptic facilitation links neuropeptides (such as cardioactive peptide SCPa and SCPb) or neurotransmitters (such as serotonin-like substances) with gating of ionic channels. Modulatory events of plastic changes in the nervous system seem therefore to be mediated by voltage and substance dependent ionic channels. Moreover, all these modifications lead to a more potent and intense reflex withdrawal.

Sensitization has been distinguished from dishabituation, the process whereby a nociceptive stimulus relieves the reflex depression produced by habituation. More recent experiments suggest that even though dishabituation and sensitization do share a common mechanism (spike broadening), another set of mechanisms is utilized in dishabituation.

Experiments performed in cell culture demonstrated that when the synapse is depressed, a process not related to K channel modulation becomes evident, and this component seems to share with the spike broadening the feature that is also driven by cAMP, but without there being any change in the duration of the action potential.

Llinas et al. (1985) suggest that Ca^{++} is crucial for transmitter availability and mobilization as well as for the events that bind the vesicle to the release site prior to esocytosis. Recent results (Gringrich and Byrne, 1985) show that short-term habituation might involve insufficient mobilization. During dishabituation, therefore, serotonin could overcome this block by removing the transmitter.

NON-ASSOCIATIVE LEARNING IN THE LEECH HIRUDO m

With the aim of further contributing to the study of cellular and molecular mechanisms in short-term plastic changes, we investigated another invertebrate model, the leech *Hirudo m*, whose nervous system is made up of segmental ganglia. Many cellular networks underlying its simple behavioral acts have already been extensively investigated.

Two behavioral acts, the shortening reflex and the swimming, were analyzed in order to establish whether:

— the short-term change mechanisms involved in non-associative learning are invariant along the phylogenetic scale;

— the neurotransmitters and neuromodulators involved in *Aplysia* play a similar role in short-term changes of alternative systems; and

— the molecular mechanism of protein phosphorylation for short-term modifications is unique or whether additional changes appear in a more complex behavioral activity. The experiments performed on the shortening reflex demonstrated that the potentiation observed during the sensitization is mediated by 5HT through the cAMP increase (Belardetti et al., 1982).

More recently we focused our attention on the swimming activity of the leeches. This behavioral act has already been extensively studied at a cellular level (Kristian et al., 1983; Stent et al., 1981). The stimulation of mechanosensory neurons leads, at the level of each segmental ganglion, to the activation of a cascade of interconnected neurons starting with the fast oscillatory neurons which excite pattern generating neurons that, by coming into contact with the dorsal and ventral motoneurons, give rise to rhythmic contraction of longitudinal and flattener muscles. In animals in which a section between the cephalic ganglion and the first segmental ganglion has been made, light tactile or low threshold electrical stimulation onto skin areas of the tail produce almost constantly a swim cycle with a predictable latency between the start of the stimulus and the onset of the response. When trains of electrical stimuli (10/sec; 1 msec; 1-1,5 V) are repetitively applied at very low frequency (1/min), a progressive increase in latency occurs (habituation).

A strong nociceptive stimulus applied along different parts of the body wall induces a brisk shortening of the latency, both in preceding delayed habituated responses (dishabituation) and in non decremented responses (sensitization). The effect persists for 30 to 60 minutes. The following series of experiments demonstrates the involvement of 5HT and cAMP in these non associative learning processes.

1. Injection of a serotonin blocking agent, methysergide (with a concentration in the body fluid of 5×10^{-4}M), prevents the behavioral dishabituation.

2. 5HT injection into the whole animal (0.2 ml of 2×10^{-4}M solution) significantly reduces latency in swimming induction in both habituated and non-habituated animals.

3. Leeches treated with the neurotoxic agent, 5,7 DHT, did not exhibit behavioral dishabituation following noxious stimuli while treatment with 6 OHDA did not affect the shortening of latency in triggering the swim.

4. The administration of Dopamine, excitatory and inhibitory aminoacids (GABA, glycine, alanine) fails to induce sensitization.

5. The role of cAMP has been tested by using an adenylate cyclase blocking agent, RMI 12330A, which blocks the decrease in latency in producing swimming by 5HT application or by nociceptive stimulation.

All the above data clearly demonstrate that 5HT, through the formation of cAMP, mediates the short-term changes underlying non-associative learning.

CELLULAR MECHANISMS OF SHORT TERM CHANGES

Modulation of the Afterhyperpolarization of Mechanosensory Neurons

We analyzed cellular and molecular events responsible for the behavioral changes observed, and detected two important mechanisms related to short-term changes. In T, P, N mechanosensory neurons the repetitive firing produces a sustained hyperpolarization (AH) that in T neurons is due to an electrogenic pump and an increase in gK whereas in P and N it is mainly due to a Ca-dependent K current. The application of 5HT induces a dose dependent depression of the AH amplitude in T neurons. The effect, which lasts more than 30 min, is reversible and is blocked by methysergide treatment.

The direct intracellular stimulation of Retzius cells (two giant serotonergic neurons located in each ganglion) mimics the reduction of AH (Belardetti et al., 1984).

Since no detectable effect was seen on AH of P and N neurons following 5HT application (Brunelli and Demontis, unpublished data) we may assume that 5HT might act by inhibiting a membrane ATPase correlated with the Na/K pump.

A series of experiments clearly demonstrates that 5HT might act through the mediation of cAMP. The AH amplitude of sensory neurons is reduced by both the intracellular injection of cAMP into T mechanosensory neurons and by the application of forskolin (an adenylate cyclase activator) in the presence of theophylline (Brunelli and Demontis, unpublished data).

On the other hand, the AH reduction following 5HT application is prevented by pretreatment with an adenylate cyclase inhibitor (RMI 12330A Merrel). Similar modulatory effects have been observed also on the AH of CA1 neurons of hippocampus (Thompson et al., 1986).

Further experiments are required to elucidate the molecular mechanism of the action of 5HT on AH and the role it plays in the plastic changes.

Modulation of Electrotonic Synapses

In addition to this novel cellular mechanism, we recently detected a further plastic change in the segmental ganglion of the leech by studying the effect of 5HT on the two giant Retzius cells (Rz). It is well known that the latter are interconnected through an electrotonic non-rectifying synapse (Eckert, 1963; Hagiwara and Morita, 1962). By inserting two microelectrodes into one Rz cell and one electrode into the other, it is possible to calculate the coupling ratio between the two cells by applying pulses of a constant current on one side of the junction. Steady state voltage will be reached in the first cell and in its follower (V1, V2). The coupling ratio will be given by $V2/V1 = K1,2$ when the potential is generated by a current on the prejunctional side.

The ratio can be related to the resistances of the circuit:

$$K1,2 = \frac{r2}{r2+rj} \qquad \text{where } r2 = \text{input resistance of the receiving cell}$$
$$\text{and } rj = \text{junctional resistance}$$

In the reverse direction we have $V1/V2 = K2,1$, that is the *attenuation factor*. The coupling ratio might therefore vary when either the input resistance or the junctional resistance changes.

Our experiments clearly demonstrated that serotonin (2×10^{-4}M) and dopamine (2×10^{-4}M) cause a long-lasting reduction in the electrotonic coupling between the two Rz, and the effect is strongly potentiated in the presence of the phosphodiesterase inhibitor IBMX (Fig. 1).

Ach (2×10^{-4}M) fails to change the coupling ratio even if this transmitter affects the input resistance activating a Cl channel.

The direct ionthophoretical injection into one of the two Rz cells of cAMP in the presence of IBMX can cause a reduction in the electrotonic strength of the synapse. This effect is highly specific because cGMP, even when pretreated with IBMX, does not change the electrical synaptic transmission. The intracellular injection of GTPγS (an activator of adenylate cyclase) causes modifications in the coupling ratio.

Perfusion of ganglia with an agonist for D1 receptor (SKF 10^{-6} M) induces a clear decrease in the coupling ratio while blocking the D2 receptor with Clebopride (1×10^{-5} M) fails to inhibit the uncoupling effect of Dopamine. The data suggest that neurotransmitters like Serotonin and Dopamine modulate the efficacy of electrical

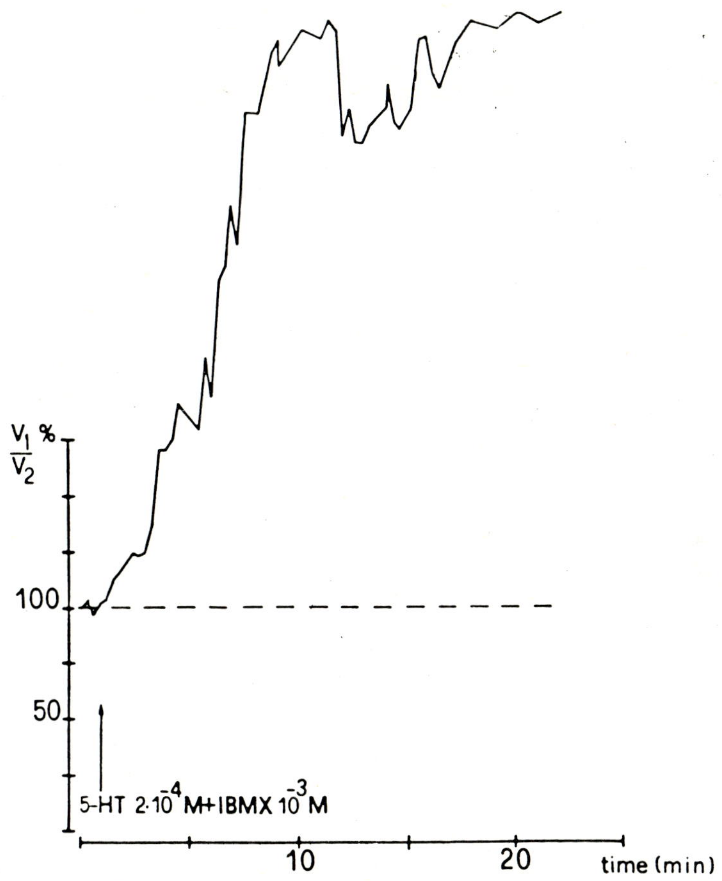

Figure 1. Uncoupling effects of 5HT and IBMX on electrotonic connection between the two Retzius cells of the leech. The graph clearly demonstrates that in a few minutes the application of 5HT (2×10^{-4}M) in the presence of the phosphodiesterase inhibitor IBMX (10^{-3}M) produces a strong and long-lasting depression of electrical synapses between the two Retzius cells. In the ordinate the coupling ratio (V_1/V_2), expressed as 100% of the control value before the neurotransmitter application. In the abscissa the time following 5HT injection.

synapses through the cyclic nucleotide increase. The effect appears to depend upon a real change in junctional permeability.

However, it is not yet known whether this effect of modulation of the gap junction following the application of neurotransmitters is limited to specific synapses or is widespread, reaching many electrical synapses in the ganglion. Nor do we know whether this plastic modification is in any way correlated to non-associative learning processes of the sensitization type. Further experiments are required to elucidate these points.

LONG-TERM LEARNING PROCESS

It is well known that the retention of learned information has two major components: the so-called short-term (S.T.) memory lasting minutes to hours and long-term (L.T.) memory lasting days or weeks.

It has been experimentally demonstrated that inhibitors of protein synthesis may disrupt the long-term changes, leaving the short-term ones unchanged, and this occurs when the inhibitors are applied 1 to 2 hours after training. But in earlier experiments of

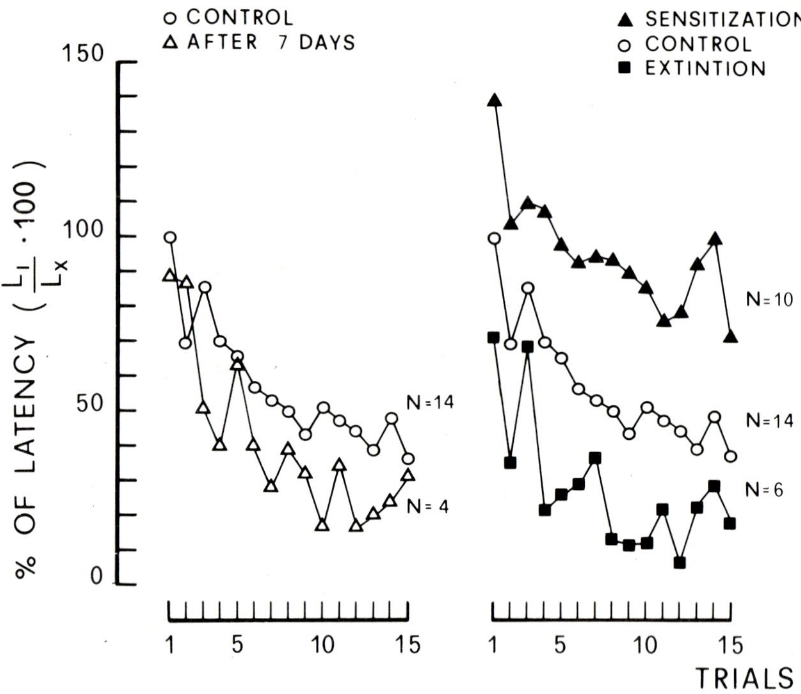

Figure 2. Long-term sensitization in the leech. In both the experimental and control groups a cut was made between the first segmental and the head ganglion. In these animals, the swimming activity was induced by light electrical stimulation of the tail. The interval between the onset of the stimulus and the beginning of the response, detected by a photocell and recorded in a polygraph, was taken as the latency in inducing swim. In the ordinate the measurements of the inverse recorded latency are shown. The first response is considered as 100%. In the curves on the left the responses of swim induction in animal group not receiving sensitizing stimuli are reported. On the first day repetitive stimuli (1/min.) produced a progressive delay in latency (habituation) (white circles). After 7 days the animals were retested again (white triangles). The two curves clearly overlap. The curves on the right report the results obtained in animals receiving daily sensitizing stimuli. The graph with white circles is the record made on the first day, while the graph with triangles is the record made on the 7th day, after six days of sensitization. The curve is statistically higher than that of the control. The curve with black squares is a recording made 5 days after terminating sensitizing stimulation. There is a clear recovery from the long-term potentiation.

this type, the inhibitors were given in systems in which it was difficult both to make an analysis at the cellular level and to compare the effects on short-term and long-term modifications.

In order to study the putative mechanisms responsible for transforming the S.T. into the L.T. processes, we devised experiments on L.T. sensitization in the behavioral model of swimming in the leech *H. medicinalis*. An L.T. habituation was obtained by applying a daily session of S.T. habituation for at least 6 days.

Likewise, it was possible to induce an L.T. sensitization with the application of one session of nociceptive stimulation every day for 6 days (Fig. 2). The experimental group presented a latency in inducing swimming that was markedly lower than that of the untreated control group and than that measured on the first day. This latency potentiation lasted for several days after which gradual return to normal latency was observed.

We obtained also an L.T. sensitization by daily injecting the animals with 5 HT. We observed an L.T. potentiation by a massive training through the application, at regular intervals for 24 hours, of the same amounts of stimuli given over 6 days. The S.T. potentiation (dishabituation) induced in the experimental group in the first day was of the same amplitude as that obtained the last day.

When applied on alternate days, inhibitors of protein synthesis (Cycloheximide), selectively blocked the L.T. facilitation of inducing swimming whereas the S.T. modifications were unchanged, indicating:
— that S.T. and L.T. memory exhibit different mechanisms and
— that L.T. sensitization requires the formation of new protein.

This is confirmed by the fact that the L.T. sensitization is also blocked by applying every two days inhibitors of messenger RNA (Actinomycina D). Surprisingly, the L.T. habituation was not affected either by protein synthesis inhibitors or by mRNA inhibitors.

These data are in accordance with recent findings made by Montarolo et al., 1986. In the cultured neurons which mediate the withdrawal reflex of *Aplysia*, the authors observed that protein synthesis inhibitors block the L.T. potentiation of the EPSP recorded in motoneurons after sensory neurons stimulation.

CONCLUSIONS

The mechanisms of short- and long-term plastic changes underlying the non-associative type of learning process are summarized in Figure 3.

Neurotransmitters or neuromodulators might trigger a cascade of events leading to:
— adenylate cyclase complex activation;
— increase in endogenous cAMP;
— protein kinase activation;
— phosphorylation of proteins; and
— gating of ionic channels such as Ks closure.

This scheme is valid for many invertebrate models (*Aplysia, Hermissenda, Hirudo*) and clearly indicates that in S.T. memory there is only a change in the preexisting protein

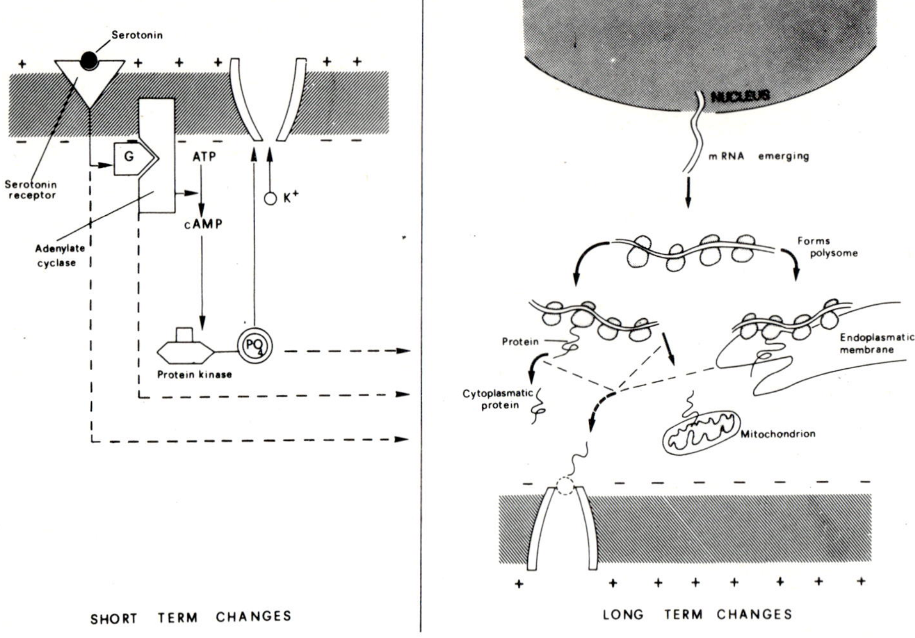

Figure 3. Diagram illustrating the chain of events leading to the short- and long-term modifications underlying behavioral sensitization. 5HT triggers the short-term changes through a mechanism of cAMP dependent protein phosphorylation, while the long-term changes seem due to the synthesis of a new protein.

by means of a process of cAMP dependent phosphorylation. The S.T. process might be sustained by Ca/calmodulin phosphorylated proteins.

Recent experiments performed in our laboratories have characterized the substrate of some cAMP and CA/calmodulin dependent protein kinases in ganglia homogenates as well as in intact ganglia. It has yet to be clarified which of these proteins is involved in the learning processes.

Figure 3 also shows the mechanism that might be responsible for the transformation from short- to long-term learning. A trigger may originate from different sources, either from neurotransmitter binding sites, from cyclase or from protein kinase activation, and this trigger in neurons would induce the formation of new proteins from different intracellular sites. The proteins might persistently affect the ionic channel gating. In favor of this hypothesis is a recent report by Scholtz and Byrne (1987), who observe that a voltage clamp analysis of the sensory neurons controlling the reflex in *Aplysia*, 24 hours after sensitization training, reveals a significant reduction in net outward current.

As yet we do not know whether the newly formed protein is directly responsible for the modulation of ionic channels or whether it is an intermediate trigger leading to a further chain of events.

It therefore seems likely that L.T. memory is induced by a chain of intracellular processes leading to the formation of substances which might provide the storage of information for a prolonged period of time.

REFERENCES

Belardetti F, Biondi C, Brunelli M, Colombaioni L, Trevisani A(1982) Role of serotonin and CAMP on facilitation of the first conducting system activity in the Hirudo medicinalis. Brain Res 246: 89-103.

Belardetti F, Brunelli M, Demontis G, Sonetti D (1984) Serotonin and Retzius cell depress the hyperpolarization following impulses of leech touch cell. Brain Res 300: 91-102.

Brunelli M, Castellucci VF, Kandel ER (1976) Synaptic facilitation and behavioral sensitization in Aplysia: possible role of serotonin and CAMP. Science 194: 1178-1181.

Eckert R (1963) Electrical interaction of paired ganglion cells in the leech. J Gen Physiol 46: 573-588.

Gringrich KS, Byrne JH (1985) Stimulation of synaptic depression posttetanic potentiation, and presynaptic facilitation of synaptic potentials from sensory neurons mediating gill withdrawal reflex in Aplysia. J Neurophysiol 53: 652-660.

Hagiwara S, Morita H (1962) Electrotonic transmission between two nerve cells in leech ganglion. J Neurophysiol 25: 721-731.

Kandel ER, Schwartz JH (1982) Molecular biology of learning: modulation of transmitter release. Science 218: 433-443.

Kristan W (1983) The neurobiology of swimming in the leech. Trends in Neuroscience 6: 84-89.

Llinas R, McGuiness TL, Leonard CS, Sugimori M, Greengard P (1985) Intraterminal injection of synapse I or Calcium/Calmodulin dependent protein kinase II alters neurotransmitter release at squid giant synapse. Proc Natl Acad Sci USA 82: 3035-3039.

Stent G, Kristan W (1981) Neural circuits generating rhythmic movements. Neurobiology of the leech. In: Cold Spring Harbor Laboratory, pp. 113-146.

Thompson SM, Prince DA (1986) Activation of electrogenic pump in hippocampal CA_1 neurons following glutamate-induced depolarization. J Neurophysiol 56: 507-522.

Plenary Lecture on:
RESEARCH STRATEGIES
FOR THE THERAPY OF AGING BRAIN

Giancarlo Pepeu
Professor of Pharmacology
University of Florence

Neuronal Plasticity and Trophic Factors
G. Biggio, P.F. Spano, G. Toffano, S.H. Appel, G.L. Gessa (eds.)
Fidia Research Series, Symposia in Neuroscience VII
Liviana Press, Padova © 1988

RESEARCH STRATEGIES FOR THE THERAPY OF AGING BRAIN

Giancarlo Pepeu and Ileana Marconcini Pepeu

Department of Preclinical and Clinical Pharmacology, University of Florence,
Viale Morgagni 65, 50134 Florence, Italy

The term "aging brain" includes several physiological and pathological conditions, listed in Table 1, which only have in common the occurrence after 65 years of age, the conventional beginning of old age. Parkinson's disease could also be considered an aspect of aging brain, but the strategies for its treatment are well established (Yahr, 1986) and will not be discussed here.

Of the four conditions listed in Table 1, Alzheimer's disease (AD) is considered the most severe and, using the words of the President of the United States, "the emotional, financial and social consequences of Alzheimer's disease are so devastating that it deserves special attention" (U.S. Department of Health and Human Services, Report, 1984).

Examining postmortem histological changes, Tomlinson et al. (1970) found that AD represents 56% of all cases of dementia while 18% are the cases of multinfarct dementia and 18% the mixed forms. The remaining 8% showed no abnormality or other specific dementias. The prevalence ratio for AD ranges between 1.2 and 5.8 cases per 100 population aged 65 and over (Rocca et al., 1986).

Multinfarct dementia is a well defined clinical entity and its diagnosis can be made using a series of standard clinical parameters (Loeb, 1980). Its frequency of association with deep white matter changes, recently called "leuko-araiosis" by Hachinski et al. (1987), is stronger than in other forms of dementia (Inzitari et al., 1987). Possibilities of

---

Abbreviations: ACh: acetylcholine, AD: Alzheimer's disease, ChAT: choline acetyltransferase, GM1: GM1 monosialoganglioside, NGF: nerve growth factor.

confusion between AD and multinfarct dementia still remain, however, as shown by the fairly large group of mixed forms.

The fourth condition listed in Table 1 is the "age-associated memory impairment", a term which is substituting the previous "benign senescent forgetfulness" (Kral, 1962) and indicates the decline in the ability to remember certain types of information which occurs in many healthy individuals during the later decades of adult life (Crook et al., 1986). There is a large and growing amount of literature describing the psychobiological changes associated with memory decline in aging (Zornetzer, 1986; Winblad et al., 1985; Flicker et al., 1985). Age-related memory impairment also occurs in animals (Bartus et al., 1978; Ingram 1985) and remarkable analogies between memory deficits in aging monkeys and men have been demonstrated on a delayed response task (Dean and Bartus, 1985).

Table 1. *Definition of aging brain*

1. Senile dementia (of Alzheimer and Alzheimer's type)
2. Multinfarct dementia
3. Mixed forms
4. Age-associated memory impairment

However, the borderline between "normal" memory loss and pathological loss during aging is not always clear and the finding of Steingart et al. (1987) that leuco-araiosis is present in 9 out of 105 "normal" elderly volunteers showing a lower score at psychometric evaluation leaves open the question on how "normal" the age-related memory impairment is.

The main target of research should therefore be the therapy of AD without disregarding the possibility of obtaining an improvement of the age-associated memory impairment.

The strategies through which drugs for incurable diseases were discovered in the past are two: serendipity and rational planning based on knowledge of the causes and pathogenetic mechanisms. If serendipity means, according to Horatio Walpole and the Oxford Dictionary, "making discoveries by accident and sagacity of things (one is) not in quest of", the antipsychotics and antidepressants are examples of important drugs discovered by serendipity. Chlorpromazine, the first antipsychotic, was synthesized as an antihistaminic and imipramine, the first tricyclic antidepressant, was synthetized as an antipsychotic (Snyder, 1986). On the contrary, the treatment of Parkinson's disease with 1-Dopa was the rational consequence of the discovery that the lack of dopamine in the striatum was an important pathogenetic factor of this disease (Hornykiewicz, 1973).

While we wait for research to come out with a serendipitous discovery for AD therapy, a rational approach must rely on the following conditions: knowledge of etiology or at least pathogenetic mechanisms and availability of animal models.

The etiology of AD is far from being understood. There is evidence for a genetic component in AD (Davies, 1987). The genetic defect has been localized on chromosome 21 but its link with the gene for beta amyloid production is doubtful (Tanzi et al., 1987). These discoveries are very important and open the way to genetic counseling but do not offer yet a lead for pharmacological intervention. The immunological and viral hypotheses of AD are not supported by evidence strong enough to warrant therapeutic approaches.

The main pathogenetic factors involved in the complex picture of AD are listed in Table 2.

Table 2. *Pathogenetic factors of Alzheimer's disease*

Plaque and neurofibrillary tangle formation
Neuron loss
Neurotransmitter decrease

PLAQUES AND FIBRILLARY TANGLES FORMATION

Information is beginning to become available on the composition, chemical and immunological properties of the amyloid beta protein found in the senile plaques, cerebrovascular amyloid deposits and neurofibrillary tangles of AD patients (Selkoe, 1987). The mechanisms of its formation are still elusive. Nevertheless, the possibility can be envisaged that the abnormal synthesis of this peptide might be controlled by specific protein synthesis inhibitors. Much investigation is still needed, however, to make this approach fruitful.

NEURONAL LOSS

A small but significant neuronal loss, probably caused by the development of intracytoplasmatic fibrillary tangles, has been described in many regions of the brain in AD patients. This is associated with an exaggeration of the loss of dendrites which also occurs in normal elderly (Terry, 1980). The basal forebrain cholinergic system and the hippocampus are the regions in which the neuronal degeneration and death are more pronounced (Mani et al., 1986; Price, 1986). It has been suggested that a lack of trophic factors in aging and AD might be responsible for the neuronal degeneration although no direct demonstration has as yet been provided (Hefty and Weiner, 1986). Nevertheless, the intracerebroventricular administration of nerve growth factor (NGF) has been shown in the rat to promote the survival of septal neurons after fimbria transection (Hefti, 1986) and partly reverse the cholinergic cell body atrophy and improve retention of a spatial memory task in behaviourally impaired aged rats (Fisher et al., 1987).

Prevention of age-related cholinergic and dendritic spine loss in the basal forebrain nuclei and hippocampus, quantified by morphometric analysis in 27-month-old rats, can also be obtained by administering phosphatidylserine in the drinking water from the age of 15 months (Milan et al., 1986; Milan et al., 1987). Phosphatidylserine administration of comparable duration in man is certainly not feasible. These results, however, indicate that the age-related structural changes can be partly reversed by drug treatment.

NEURONAL PLASTICITY

On the basis of the previous findings, the hypothesis can be put forward that NGF and phosphatidylserine may enhance the neuronal plasticity which is responsible in the formation of synaptic connections and the maintenance of the integrity of the neuronal network (Freed et al., 1985). Examples of spontaneous compensatory neuronal plasticity can be found in AD patients. Geddes et al. (1985) observed a spontaneous regeneration in the dentate girus molecular layer in hippocampal postmortem samples. Arendt et al. (1986) saw an increase in the size of cell soma and degree of dendritic arborization in the diagonal band and nucleus basalis.

The possibility of stimulating the spontaneous plasticity by drug administration is supported by experiments with the monosialoganglioside GM1. Casamenti et al. (1985) demonstrated that GM1 administration for 22 days facilitates the recovery of choline acetyltransferase (ChAT) activity and conditioned response acquisition in rats with a lesion of the nucleus basalis. The recovery in ChAT activity is associated with that of ACh release from the cerebral cortex (Florian et al., 1987). Cuello et al. (1986) reported that 30 days administration of GM1 prevented the retrograde degeneration of the cholinergic neurons of the nucleus basalis in decorticated rats. There are no clinical demonstrations that these effects can be also obtained in man and it is also possible that the reduced plasticity of aging brain may prevent GM1 from exerting its action. Nevertheless, GM1, other gangliosides and trophic factors offer another research approach to aging brain treatment.

NEUROTRANSMITTER DECREASE

After the first observation of Davies and Maloney (1976) that in postmortem brains of subjects affected by AD there was a considerable loss of ChAT, particularly in the hippocampus and temporal cortex, a decrease in many other neurotransmitters has been reported. According to the reviews of Gottfries (1985), Hardy et al. (1985) and Rossor and Iversen (1986), together with a reduced ACh formation there is a decrease in noradrenaline, dopamine, serotonin, GABA, somatostatin, substance P.

Great importance is still given, for two reasons, to the cholinergic deficit and several strategies have been devised for correcting it. First, the reduction in presynaptic markers for cholinergic transmission is the most consistent neurochemical change in AD; second, a relationship between both intellectual impairment, the amount of pathological abnormalities and the loss of ChAT in autopsy and biopsy samples has been demonstrated (Perry et al., 1978; Wilcock et al., 1982). Furthermore, lesion of the nucleus basalis in the rat mimics some of the neurochemical and cognitive impairment of AD thus presenting a useful animal model (Pepeu et al., 1986). It was initially hoped, therefore, that, as in Parkinson's disease where dopamine deficit can be corrected by the administration of the precursor lDOPA, in AD the deficit in ACh might be corrected by the administration of the precursor choline.

The list of the drugs currently proposed for correcting the cholinergic deficit is reported in Table 3. The results obtained with these drugs are summarized by Crook (1985). More than 20 controlled studies with choline and lecithin make it possible to

Table 3. *Drugs proposed for the cholinergic deficit*

Acetylcholine precursors:
— Choline
— Phosphatidylcholine (lecithin)

Acetylcholinesterase inhibitors:
— Physostigmine
— Tetrahydroaminoacridine (THA)

Muscarinic agonists:
— Arecoline
— Betanechol
— RS 86

conclude that precursor therapy is not an effective treatment in AD. Trials with anticholinesterase inhibitors and muscarinic agonists are somewhat more encouraging, and clinally modest but quite clear drug effects on selected cognitive measures have been obtained in some AD patients.

Animal studies demonstrate that other drugs are able to activate brain cholinergic mechanisms and could be useful for correcting the cholinergic deficit in the aging brain. 4-aminopyridine and its derivatives strongly stimulate ACh release through the blockade of K^+ channels (Casamenti et al., 1982). Unfortunately, the toxicity of these compounds is high. It has been shown that it is possible to restore the age-dependent decrease in ACh release observed in electrically stimulated cortical slices prepared from aging rats by a 7 days treatment with phosphatidylserine (Vannucchi and Pepeu, 1987). Phosphatidylserine treatment has also been shown to improve learning and memory in aging rats (Corwin et al., 1985). The cognition-enhancing agent oxiracetam prevents the amnesia and decrease in brain ACh induced by electroconvulsive shocks or scopolamine in the rats (Spignoli and Pepeu, 1986; Spignoli and Pepeu, 1987). The toxicity of the latter two drugs is remarkably low and the clinical results in AD patients (SMID, 1987; Villardita et al., 1987) are at least as good as those obtained with cholinesterase inhibitors and muscarinic agonists. The question remains open as to whether the clinical activity depends on their action on brain cholinergic mechanisms or on other mechanisms and further trials are needed in order to fully evaluate their clinical usefulness.

MULTINFARCT DEMENTIA

Multinfarct dementia has vascular origin and a strong association with hypertension, history of stroke and signs of arteriosclerosis (Inzitari et al., 1987; Loeb, 1980). Histological changes reminiscent of multinfarct dementia, associated with a modest cognitive and psychomotor impairment, can be seen in the brain of spontaneously hypertensive rats (Banfi and Dorigotti, 1986). Strategies for the therapy of multinfarct dementia must therefore be mostly preventive removing the cardiovascular pathology that will eventually bring about dementia. Experimental

(Banfi and Dorigotti, 1986) and clinical evidence (Moglia et al., 1986) indicates that cognition-enhancing agents may ameliorate the cognitive and psychomotor deficits, once they are established.

CRITERIA FOR SELECTING A DRUG FOR THE AGING BRAIN

Attempts to ameliorate AD and age-dependent memory impairment are not confined only to the administration of drugs acting on brain cholinergic system. The strategy based on replacement of neurotransmitters of which a decrease in AD patients has been reported has led to the administration of 1-DOPA, tryptophan and inhibitors of serotonin uptake (Gottfries, 1985). The results, when present, are modest and of little clinical utility. In addition, outside of the neurotransmitter realm, the list of drugs which are currently used or under trial for the aging brain, including AD, is very long (Crook, 1985; Allain et al., 1986) but their clinical utility is always limited. Facing this not very optimistic situation, the rational selection of new drugs or the evaluation of old drugs for aging brain should always be guided by few criteria which are neither new nor original, but are frequently forgotten. According to them, a potentially useful drug should have:
— effect on the pathogenetic mechanism if not on the etiology;
— activity on animal models (aging animals, animals with specific lesions);
— low toxicity (unless it is a miracle drug); and
— easy route of administration.

The question remains open as to which of the many drugs presently proposed for the therapy of aging brain corresponds to these criteria.

REFERENCES

Allain H, Reymann JM, Bentue-Ferrer D, van den Driessche J (1986) Pharmacological aspects of brain aging and dementia. In: Courtois Y, Faucheux B, Forette B, Knook DL, Trèton JA (eds): Modern trends in aging research. John Libbey Eurotext, London, pp. 473-484.

Arendt T, Zvegintseva HG, Leontovich TA (1986) Dendritic changes in the basal nucleus of Meynert and in the diagonal band nucleus in Alzheimer's disease - A quantitative Golgi investigation. Neuroscience 19:1265-1278.

Banfi S, Dorigotti L (1986) Experimental behavioral studies with oxiracetam on different types of chronic cerebral impairment. Clin Neuropharmacol 9 (suppl 3): S19-S26.

Casamenti F, Corradetti R, Löffelholz K, Mantovani P (1982) Effects of 4-aminopyridine on acetylcholine output from the cerebral cortex of the rat in vivo. Br J Pharmac 76: 439-445.

Casamenti F, Bracco L, Bartolini L, Pepeu G (1985) Effects of ganglioside treatment in rats with a lesion of the cholinergic forebrain nuclei. Brain Res 338:45-52.

Corwin J, Dean RL, Bartus RT, Rotrosen J, Watkins DL (1985) Behavioral effects of phosphatidylserine in the aged Fisher 344 rats: amelioration of passive avoidance deficits without changes in psychomotor task performance. Neurobiol Aging 6:11-15.

Crook T (1985) Clinical drug trials in Alzheimer's disease. In: Olton DS, Gamzu E, Corkin S (eds): Memory dysfunctions: an integration of animal and human research from preclinical to clinical perspectives. Ann N Y Acad Sci 444:428-436.

Crook T, Bartus RT, Ferris S, Whitehouse P, Cohen GD, Gershon S (1986) Age-associated memory impairment: proposed diagnostic criteria and measures of clinical change. Devel Neuropsychol 4:425-437.

Cuello AC, Stephens PH, Tagari PC, Sofroniew MV, Pearson RCA (1986) Retrograde changes in the nucleus basalis of the rat, caused by cortical damage, are prevented by exogenous ganglioside GM1. Brain Res 376:373-377.

Davies P (1987) The genetic of Alzheimer's disease: a review and a discussion of the implications. Neurobiol Aging 7:459-466.

Dean RL, Bartus RT (1985) Animal models of geriatric cognitive dysfunction: evidence for an important cholinergic involvement. In: Traber J, Gispen WG (eds): Senile dementia of the Alzheimer's type. Springer Verlag, Berlin, pp. 269-282.

Fisher W, Wictorin K, Bjorklund A, William LR, Varon S, Gage FH (1987) Amelioration of cholinergic neuron atrophy and spatial memory impairment in aged rats by nerve growth factor. Nature 329:65-68.

Flicker C, Ferris SH, Crook T, Bartus RT, Reisberg B (1985) Cognitive function in normal aging and early dementia. In: Traber J, Gispen WG (eds): Senile dementia of the Alzheimer's type. Springer Verlag, Berlin, pp. 2-17.

Florian A, Casamenti F, Pepeu G (1987) Recovery of cortical acetylcholine output after ganglioside treatment in rats with lesion of the nucleus basalis. Neurosci Lett 75:313-316.

Freed WJ, de Medinaceli L, Wyatt RJ (1985) Promoting functional plasticity in the damaged nervous system. Science 227:1544-1552.

Geddes W, Monaghan DT, Cotman CW, Lott IT, Kim RC, Chang Chui H (1985) Plasticity of hippocampal circuitry in Alzheimer's disease. Science 230:1179-1181.

Gottfries CG (1985) Alzheimer's disease and senile dementia: biochemical characteristics and aspect of treatment. Psychopharmacol 86:245-252.

Guidolin D, Milan F, Polato P, Nunzi MG, Toffano G (1987) Phosphatidylserine treatment prevents age-induced structural alterations in the rat septo-hippocampal system. In: Bazan NG, Horrocks L, Toffano G (eds): Phospholipids in the nervous system: biochemical and molecular pathology. Liviana, Padova, in press.

Hachinski VC, Potter P, Merskey H (1987) Leuko-araiosis. Arch Neurol 44:21-23.

Hardy J, Adolsson R, Alafuzoff I, Bucht G, Marcusson J, Nyberg P, Perdhal E, Wester P, Winblad B (1985) Transmitter deficits in Alzheimer's disease. Neurochem Int 7:545-563.

Hefti F (1986) Nerve growth factor (NGF) promotes survival of septal cholinergic neurons after fimbrial transections. J Neurosci 6:2155-2162.

Hefti F, Weiner WJ (1986) Nerve growth factor and Alzheimer's disease. Ann Neurol 20:275-281.

Hornykiewicz O (1973) Parkinson's disease: from brain homogenate to treatment. Fed Proc 32:183-190.

Ingram DK (1985) Analysis of age-related impairments in learning and memory in rodent models. In: Olton DS, Gamzu E, Corkin S (eds): Memory dysfunctions: an integration of animal and human research from preclinical to clinical perspectives. Ann N Y Acad Sci 444:312-331.

Inzitari D, Diaz F, Fox A, Hachinski VC, Steingart A, Lau C, Wade DJ, Mulic H, Merskey H (1987) Vascular risk and leuko-araiosis. Arch Neurol 44:42-47.

Loeb C (1980) Clinical diagnosis of multinfarct dementia. In: Amaducci L, Davison AN, Antuono P (eds): Aging of the brain and dementia. Raven Press, New York, pp. 251-260.

Many RB, Lohr JB, Jeste DV (1986) Hippocampal pyramidal cells and aging in the human: a quantitative study of neuronal loss in sector CA1 to CA4. Exptl Neurol 94:29-40.

Milan F, Nunzi MG, Guidolin D, Calderini G, Toffano G (1986) Age-related loss of dendritic spines in rat hippocampus: effect of phosphatidylserine administration. In: Bes A, Cahn J, Cahn R, Hoyer S, Marc-Vergnes JP, Wisniewski MM (eds): Senile dementia: early detection. John Libbey Eurotext, London, pp. 408-413.

Moglia A, Sinforiani E, Zandrini C, Gualtieri S, Corsico R, Arrigo A (1986) Activity of oxiracetam in patients with organic brain syndrome: a neuropsychological study. Clin Neuropharmacol 9 (suppl 3): S73-78.

Pepeu G, Casamenti F, Pedata F, Cosi C, Marconcini Pepeu I (1986) Are the neurochemical and behavioral changes induced by lesions of the nucleus basalis in the rat a model of Alzheimer's disease? Neuro-Psychopharmacol & Biol Psychiat 10: 541-551.

Perry EK, Tomlinson BE, Blessed G, Bergman K, Gibson PH, Perry RH (1978) Correlation of cholinergic abnormalities with senile plaques and mental test score in senile dementia. Br Med J 2:1457-1459.

Price DL (1986) New perspectives on Alzheimer's disease. Ann Rev Neurosci 9:489-512.

Rocca WA, Amaducci A, Schoenberg BS (1986) Epidemiology of clinically diagnosed Alzheimer's disease. Ann Neurol 19:415-424.

Rossor M, Iversen LL (1986) Non-cholinergic neurotransmitter abnormalities in Alzheimer's disease. Br Med Bull 42:70-74.

SMID Group (1987) Phosphatidylserine in the treatment of clinically diagnosed Alzheimer's disease. In: Wurtman RJ, Corkin SH, Growdon JH (eds): Alzheimer's disease: advanced in basic research and therapies. Center for Brain Sciences and Metabolism Charitable Trusts, Cambridge, pp. 305-314.

Snyder S (1986) Drugs and the brain. Scientific American Books, New York.

Spignoli G, Pepeu G (1986) Oxiracetam prevents electroshock-induced decrease in brain acetylcholine and amnesia. Eur J Pharmacol 126:253-257.

Spignoli G, Pepeu G (1987) Interactions between oxiracetam, aniracetam and scopolamine on behavior and brain acetylcholine. Pharmacol Biochem Behav 27:491-495.

Steingart A, Hachinski VC, Lau C, Fox AJ, Diaz F, Cape R, Lee D, Inzitari D, Merskey H (1987) Cognitive and neurological findings in subjects with diffuse white matter lucencies on computed tomographic scan (Leuko-araiosis). Arch Neurol 44:32-39.

Tanzi RE, St George-Hilsop PH, Haines JL, Polinsky RJ, Nee L, Foncin JF, Neve RL, McClatchey AI, Coneally PM, Gusella JM (1987) The genetic defect in familial Alzheimer's disease is not tightly linked to the amyloid beta protein gene. Nature 329:156-157.

Terry RD Structural changes in senile dementia of the Alzheimer's type (1980) In: Amaducci L, Davison AN, Antuono P (eds): Aging of the brain and dementia. Raven Press, New York, pp. 23-32.

Tomlinson BE, Blessed G, Roth M (1970) Observations on the brain of demented old people. J Neurol Sci 11:205-242.

U.S. Department of Health and Human Sciences (1984) Report of the Secretary Task Force on Alzheimer's Disease. U.S. Government Printing Office, Washington.

Villardita C, Parini J, Grioli S, Quattropani M, Lomeo C, Scapagnini U (1987) Clinical and neuropsychological study with oxiracetam versus placebo in mild to moderate dementia patients. In: Wurtman RJ, Corkin SH, Growdon JH (eds): Alzheimer's disease: advanced in basic research and therapies. Center for Brain Sciences and Metabolism Charitable Trusts, Cambridge, pp. 619-624.

Wilcock GF, Esiri MM, Bowen DM, Smith CCT (1982) Alzheimer's disease: correlation of cortical choline acetyltransferase activity with the severity of dementia and histological abnormalities. J Neurol Sci 57:407-417.

Winblad B, Hardy J, Backman L, Nilsson LG (1985) Memory function and brain biochemistry in normal aging and senile dementia. In: Oldon D, Gamzu E, Corkin S (eds): Memory dysfunctions: an integration of animal and human research from preclinical to clinical perspectives. Ann N Y Acad Sci 444:255-268.

Yahr MD (ed) (1986) Parkinsonism: current perspectives and new horizons. Clin Neuropharmacol 9 (suppl 1).

Zornetzer SF (1986) Applied aspect of memory research: aging. In: Martinez JL, Kesner RP (eds): Learning and memory. A biological view. Academic Press, Orlando, pp. 203-233.

CONTRIBUTORS

A.J. Aguayo
Neurosciences Unit, The Montreal General Hospital and McGill University, 1650 Cedar Avenue, Montreal, H3G 1A4, Quebec, Canada

S.H. Appel
Department of Neurology, Baylor College of Medicine, Texas Medical Center, Houston, Texas 77030, U.S.A.

C.E. Bandtlow
Max-Planck Institute for Psychiatry, Dept. of Neurochemistry, Am Klopferspitz 18a, D-8033 Planegg-Martinsried, FRG

D. Benvegnú
FIDIA Research Laboratories, Via Ponte della Fabbrica, 3/A, 35031 Abano Terme, Italy

M. Blaber
Department of Biological Chemistry, California College of Medicine, University of California, Irvine, CA 92717, U.S.A.

J.R. Bostwick
Department of Neurology, Baylor College of Medicine, Houston, Texas 77030, U.S.A.

R.A. Bradshaw
Department of Biological Chemistry, California College of Medicine, University of California, Irvine, CA 92717, U.S.A.

G.M. Bray
Neurosciences Unit, The Montreal General Hospital and McGill University, 1650 Cedar Avenue, Montreal, H3G 1A4, Quebec, Canada

M. Brunelli
Department of Physiology and Biochemistry, University of Pisa, Via S. Zeno, 31, 56100 Pisa, Italy

P. Calissano
Institute of Neurobiology, CNR, Via Romagnosi 18/A, 00196 Roma, Italy

L. Callegaro
FIDIA Research Laboratories, Via Ponte della Fabbrica, 3/A, 35031 Abano Terme, Italy

K. Cavanaugh
Department of Biological Chemistry, California College of Medicine, University of California, Irvine, CA 92717, U.S.A.

M.T. Ciotti
Institute of Neurobiology, CNR, Via Romagnosi 18/A, 00196 Roma, Italy

L. Colombaioni
Department of Physiology and Biochemistry, University of Pisa, Via S. Zeno, 31, 56100 Pisa, Italy

A.C. Cuello
Department of Pharmacology and Therapeutics, McIntyre Medical Science Building, McGill University, Montreal PQ, Quebec, Canada, H3G 1Y6

R. Dal Toso
FIDIA Research Laboratories, Via Ponte della Fabbrica, 3/A, 35031 Abano Terme, Italy

A.M. Davies
St. George's Hospital Medical School, Dept. of Anatomy, London SW17 ORE, UK

J. Eldridge
Laboratory of Biochemistry, National Cancer Institute, National Institutes of Health, Bethesda MD 20892, U.S.A.

D.D. Eveleth
Department of Biological Chemistry, California College of Medicine, University of California, Irvine, CA 92717, U.S.A.

N. Ferrara
Cancer Research Institute, M-1282, University of California Medical Center, 3rd Parnasse Avenue, San Francisco, CA 94143, California, U.S.A.

G. Ferrari
FIDIA Research Laboratories, Via Ponte della Fabbrica, 3/A, 35031 Abano Terme, Italy

D. Garofalo
Department of Pharmacology and Therapeutics, McIntyre Medical Science Building, McGill University, Montreal PQ, Quebec, Canada, H3G 1Y6

D. Gospodarowicz
Cancer Research Institute, M-1282, University of California Medical Center, 3rd Parnasse Avenue, San Francisco, CA 94143, California, U.S.A.

L.A. Greene
Laboratory of Cellular and Molecular Neurobiology, Department of Pathology, Columbia University College of Physicians and Surgeons, New York, NY 10032, U.S.A.

L.J. Haverkamp
Department of Neurology, Baylor College of Medicine, Texas Medical Center, Houston, Texas 77030, U.S.A.

R. Heumann
Max-Planck Institute for Psychiatry, Dept of Neurochemistry, Am Kopferspitz 18a, D-8033 Planegg-Martinsried, FRG

P.J. Isackson
Department of Biological Chemistry, Anatomy and Neurobiology, California College of Medicine, University of California, Irvine, CA 92717, U.S.A.

H.I. Kornblum
Department of Pharmacology, California College of Medicine, University of California, Irvine CA 92717, U.S.A.

S. Korsching
California Institute of Technology, Division of Biology 216-76, Pasadena, CA 91125, U.S.A.

A. Leon
FIDIA Research Laboratories, Via Ponte della Fabbrica, 3/A, 35031 Abano Terme, Italy

F. Leslie
Department of Pharmacology, California College of Medicine, University of California, Irvine, CA 92717, U.S.A.

A. Levi
Institute of Neurobiology, CNR, Via Romagnosi 18a, 00196 Roma, Italy

I. Marconcini-Pepeu
Department of Preclinical and Clinical Pharmacology, University of Florence, Viale Morgagni 65, 50134 Florence, Italy

D. Maysinger
Department of Pharmacology and Therapeutics, McIntyre Medical Science Building, McGill University, Montreal PQ, Quebec, Canada, H3G 1Y6

J.L. McManaman
Department of Neurology, Baylor College of Medicine, Texas Medical Center, Houston, Texas 77030, U.S.A.

D. Mercanti
Institute of Neurobiology, CNR, Via Romagnosi 18/A, 00196 Roma, Italy

R.S. Morrison
Department of Neurological Surgery, Montefiore Hospital, Bronx, NY 10467, U.S.A.

B.M. Paterson
Laboratory of Biochemistry, National Cancer Institute, National Institutes of Health, Bethesda MD 20892, U.S.A.

G. Pepeu
Department of Preclinical and Clinical Pharmacology, University of Florence, Viale Morgagni 65, 50134 Florence, Italy

E.P. Pioro
Department of Pharmacology and Therapeutics, McIntyre Medical Science Building, McGill University, Montreal PQ, Quebec, Canada, H3G 1Y6

R. Possenti
Institute of Neurobiology, CNR, Via Romagnosi 18a, 00196 Roma, Italy

R.E. Rydel
Laboratory of Cellular and Molecular Neurobiology, Department of Pathology, Columbia University College of Physicians and Surgeons, New York, NY 10032, U.S.A.

M.E. Schwab
Institute of Brain Research, August-Forelstr. 1, CH-8029 Zurich, Switzerland

M. Schwarz
Department of Biological Chemistry, California College of Medicine, University of California, Irvine, CA 92717, U.S.A.

A. Sharma
Department of Physiology, California College of Medicine, University of California, Irvine, CA 92717

C. Soranzo
FIDIA Research Laboratories, Via Ponte della Fabbrica, 3/A, 35031 Abano Terme, Italy

P.C. Tagari
Department of Pharmacology and Therapeutics, McIntyre Medical Science Building, McGill University, Montreal PQ, Quebec, Canada, H3G 1Y6

H. Thoenen
Max-Planck Institute for Psychiatry, Dept. of Neurochemistry, Am Klopferspitz 18a, D-8033 Planegg-Martinsried, FRG

G. Toffano
FIDIA Research Laboratories, Via Ponte della Fabbrica, 3/A, 35031 Abano Terme, Italy

G. Traina
Department of Physiology and Biochemistry, University of Pisa, Via S. Zeno, 31, 56100 Pisa, Italy

M. Vidal-Sanz
Neurosciences Unit, The Montreal General Hospital and McGill University, 1650 Cedar Avenue, Montreal, H3G 1A4, Quebec, Canada

M.P. Villegas-Perez
Neurosciences Unit, The Montreal General Hospital and McGill University, 1650 Cedar Avenue, Montreal, H3G 1A4, Quebec, Canada

SUBJECT INDEX

Acetylcholine synthesis, 2
Aging brain, 141
Alzheimer's disease (AD), 113, 141
cAMP, 131
Anti-ChAT monoclonal antibody, 112
Anti-NGF receptor monoclonal antibody, 112
Axotomized CNS neurons, 121, 124
BHK-21 cells, 56, 69
Bovine caudate, 88
8-Br-cAMP, 74
C-CTF, 5
Central nervous system (CNS), 5, 9, 15, 105
Cerebellar granule cells, 95, 99
— adhesion, 96
— neurite outgrowth and fasciculation, 96
Choline acetyltransferase activity (ChT), 2, 108, 110, 144
Cholinergic neurons, 2
CPT-cAMP [8 (4-chlorophenylthio) cAMP], 74
Dishabituation, 129, 131, 134
Dopaminergic neurons, 88
ECM (extracellular matrix), 58, 63
EFG (epidermal growth factor), 10
— biosynthesis of, 10
— function of, 15
Embryonic rat cortical implants, 111
aFGF (acidic fibroblast growth factor), 5, 10, 53
— biological effects of, 60, 64
— mRNA, 54
bFGF (basic fibroblast growth factor), 5, 10, 53
— biological effects of, 60, 64
— biosynthesis of, 10
— function of, 16
— gene expression, 56
— mRNA, 54
FGF receptors, 59
Foetal mesencephalic cells, 88
Forebrain cholinergic neurons, 105, 111
— retrograde degeneration of, 106, 113
GABAergic neurons, 88
Gangliosides, 105, 106
Gene expression, 45
GIF technique, 88
GM$_1$ (monogangliosides), 106, 108, 110, 144
Guinea pig prostata, 14

Habituation, 129, 131, 134
Heparin, 62
Hirudo medicinalis, 130
5-HT, 130, 132
Invertebrates, 129
Long-term learning process, 129, 134
Mechanosensory neurons, 131
Motor neurons, 2
Mouse submandibular gland, 10
Mouse whisker pad, 41
Multinfarct dementia, 141, 145
Neurite outgrowth adhesion factor (NOAF), 97
Neuronal loss, 143
Neuronal plasticity, 144
Neuronal survival, 74
Neurotransmitter decrease, 144
NGF (nerve growth factor), 1, 23, 35, 45, 73, 105, 110, 143
— cellular localization of synthesis, 36
— distribution of, 24
— in situ hybridization, 36
— mRNA, 24, 36
— synthesis of, 24
Nucleus basalis magnocellularis (NBM), 105, 111
Peripheral nerve grafts, 121, 122
Peripheral nervous system, 23, 35
Pheochromocytoma (PC-12) cells, 16, 45, 61
Phosphatidylserine, 143, 145
Plaques and fibrillary tangle formation, 143
Protamine sulfate, 62
Rabbit serum, 96
Rat iris, 38
Retinal ganglion cells, 123
Retzius cells, 132
Sciatic nerve, 24, 30, 42
SDNF (striatal-derived neuronotrophic factor), 87
Segmental ganglia, 130
Sensitization, 129, 131, 134
Sensory neurons, 73, 79
Short-term learning process, 129, 130
Sympathetic ganglia, 24
Sympathetic neurons, 73, 74
TGF$_B$ (transforming growth factor), 62
Uptake of ^{3}H-DA and ^{14}C-GABA, 88
VGF gene, 46

Finito di stampare
nel mese di giugno 1988
dalla tipolitografia «La Grafica & Stampa ed. s.r.l.» di Vicenza
per conto della Liviana Editrice s.p.a. di Padova